Healing
the
Traumatized
BRAIN

A JOHNS HOPKINS PRESS HEALTH BOOK

Healing

the

Traumatized
BRAIN

*Coping after
Concussion and
Other Brain Injuries*

SANDEEP VAISHNAVI, MD, PhD

VANI RAO, MBBS, MD

Foreword by Peter V. Rabins, MD, MPH

JOHNS HOPKINS UNIVERSITY PRESS

BALTIMORE

Note to the Reader*:* This book is not meant to substitute for medical care of people with brain injury, and treatment should not be based solely on its contents. Instead, treatment must be developed in a dialogue between the individual and their physician. Our book has been written to help with that dialogue.

Drug dosage: The authors and publisher have made reasonable efforts to determine that the selection of drugs discussed in this text conforms to the practices of the general medical community. The medications described do not necessarily have specific approval by the US Food and Drug Administration for use in the diseases for which they are recommended. In view of ongoing research, changes in governmental regulation, and the constant flow of information relating to drug therapy and drug reactions, the reader is urged to check the package insert of each drug for any change in indications and dosage and for warnings and precautions. This is particularly important when the recommended agent is a new and/or infrequently used drug.

© 2023 Johns Hopkins University Press
All rights reserved. Published 2023
Printed in the United States of America on acid-free paper
2 4 6 8 9 7 5 3 1

Johns Hopkins University Press
2715 North Charles Street
Baltimore, Maryland 21218
www.press.jhu.edu

Library of Congress Cataloging-in-Publication Data is available.

ISBN 978-1-4214-4661-5 (hardcover)
ISBN 978-1-4214-4662-2 (paperback)
ISBN 978-1-4214-4663-9 (ebook)

A catalog record for this book is available from the British Library.

Figures 1.2, 2.1a, 2.1b, and 3.2 are by Jacqueline Schaffer.

Special discounts are available for bulk purchases of this book. For more information, please contact Special Sales at specialsales@jh.edu.

*To our patients and caregivers,
who continuously educate us and
motivate us to do better*

Contents

PART IV. BEHAVIORAL DISORDERS CAUSED BY THE TRAUMATIZED BRAIN 133

PART V. COGNITIVE ISSUES CAUSED BY THE TRAUMATIZED BRAIN 199

PART VI. OTHER SYMPTOMS OF THE TRAUMATIZED BRAIN 245

PART VII. THE TRAUMATIZED BRAIN AND THE FUTURE 289

Foreword

In 2015 Sandeep Vaishnavi and Vani Rao published their first book, *The Traumatized Brain: A Family Guide to Understanding Mood, Memory, and Behavior after Brain Injury*. This book was among the first to detail the often-hidden effects of brain injuries on emotions, behavior, and cognition. Writing in down-to-earth language, Drs. Vaishnavi and Rao explained what steps can be taken to cope with the often-devastating changes seen after traumatic brain injuries.

Since publication of *The Traumatized Brain*, there has been dramatic progress made in our understanding of brain function, injury, and recovery. In this new book, *Healing the Traumatized Brain*, Drs. Vaishnavi and Rao show how this progress can benefit those living with brain injuries. Starting with an easily understood description of the brain and how it functions, they detail how brain injuries may lead to changes in thinking, behavior, and the ability to carry out everyday activities. Linking this information to an explanation of how the brain recovers, they then describe what can be done to maximize recovery.

Several features of *Healing the Traumatized Brain* stand out in my mind. The authors do not shy away from using medical terminology but explain these terms in ways that can help the non-professional understand what professionals mean when they use these terms. This will improve communication among the many care providers and loved ones involved in supporting the injured person. Even more important is the authors' clear ability to describe what we do and do not know.

Although much progress has been made in understanding how the brain heals, much is still unknown. Unfortunately, this knowledge gap has spurred claims and expectations that are unfounded, for example with supplements that promise to improve your memory or treatments that have no scientific basis. *Healing the Traumatized Brain* wonderfully describes what to expect, what to do to maximize recovery, and what to avoid. The authors balance this scientific approach to healing the injured brain with an empathic approach that helps appreciate the frustration of those with a brain injury and those supporting them. It is this combination of the scientific and the empathic that makes this such a special book.

PETER V. RABINS, MD, MPH
Baltimore, Maryland

Introduction

Brain injury can have many causes, including direct trauma (such as a car accident, a fall, a battle injury, or a blow to the head suffered in amateur or professional sports). This is known as a traumatic brain injury (TBI). Injury to the brain can be caused by other mechanisms, such as a brain tumor, stroke, infections, or lack of oxygen to the brain (also known as hypoxic or anoxic brain injury). Seizures can also cause brain injury or occur as a result of brain injury.

Traumatic brain injury, one of the most common types of brain injury, can be classified as mild, moderate, or severe, based on how long the person was unconscious or how long the person was in a dazed or confused state and how much time passed before they could make new memories (to learn something new and consistently remember it). Most people with mild TBI (also known as concussion) make a spontaneous recovery within the first few weeks to months after injury. But mild brain injuries are not always benign, especially if there have been multiple injuries over the years or if there are other coexisting factors (such as mental health problems, recreational drug use, misuse of prescribed medications, or poor sleep).

Each type of brain injury has its own consequences, from acute to chronic, from mild to severe. In this book, we draw on our experiences in treating people with any type of brain injury to explain what happens with these injuries. Of course, each person's experience is different, depending on many factors—the severity of injury, other injuries the person may have suffered, medical problems, medications, misuse of prescribed medications, recreational drug use, the person's personality traits, and their genetic vulnerability. We address mild as well as moderate to severe brain injuries. The common theme is our focus on long-term problems following brain injury. Although traditional thinking has been that it is moderate to severe injuries that lead to long-term problems, there is some emerging evidence that repeated mild injuries may also be associated with long-term consequences. Such repeated mild injuries may occur in the context of contact sports such as football, especially professional football, but even perhaps with amateur (school and college) football, as well as soccer, boxing, and other contact sports.

Brain injuries have a huge impact, both literally and figuratively. People with brain injury, for example, may suffer not only from the immediate consequences of the injury, such as the potential for bleeding in the brain or for seizures, but also from long-term problems, which are often related to changes in mood, thinking, attention, memory, and behavior. The long-term problems can be confusing to family and friends who may think that their loved one with brain injury has changed but be unable to understand why. These types of cognitive, emotional, and behavioral problems (often known as neuropsychiatric problems) can have a great impact on quality of life. If the problems are not recognized by the person with the brain injury and their family, misunderstandings may follow.

Brain injuries are in a sense silent, because after persons with brain injury have been treated in the emergency department or released from the hospital, family members or friends may assume that they are now healed. There may be no obvious physical evidence of injury, so it is easy for others to believe that everything is back to normal, though in reality, things may not be normal in the brain.

We spend much of the book discussing the emotional, cognitive, and behavioral problems following brain injury. Even though these problems develop after the injury, they may not always be directly related to the injury. Brain injury may be one of several contributors; other pre-injury and post-injury factors may also contribute. Persons with neuropsychiatric problems prior to injury are at risk of developing them after injury. Whatever the cause may be, these problems are often not well recognized and continue to be distressing to both the person with brain injury and their family.

The person with brain injury may not be able to function well because of emotional, cognitive, or behavioral problems, so relationships and employment suffer as the person is unable to achieve their full potential. Although a person may appear to have healed in appearance and maybe even in skills, it is not until the environment challenges them that the impact of the brain injury may emerge. It may do so in a way that those observing a related struggle might not link it to that person's history of brain injury. The person with the injury may not be able to explain, for example, why it takes them an hour to unload the dishwasher, or why they are struggling to do simple tasks that before they could have easily carried out. These outcomes are particularly tragic because many of the problems are manageable. The brain is traumatized physically by brain injury, but the event in itself can also lead to emotional trauma. Furthermore, family members themselves may be emotionally traumatized; they may not understand why their loved one has changed so much and may not know even how to begin to help.

One aim in this book is to continue to give voice to this some-times-silent injury and everyone affected by it. We want to educate and thus empower people who have suffered from brain injuries as well as their loved ones. We want to help readers recognize and understand the neuropsychiatric problems that can develop after brain injury. Unlike physical problems, such as a change in appearance or a change in one's ability to get around, neuropsychiatric problems are often overlooked or misunderstood. Recognizing these problems is the first step in addressing them. We discuss in general some of the medication treatments that have proven to be helpful. We also advise the reader on general actions to take and some behavioral methods to use to minimize neuropsychiatric problems after brain injury.

We also aim to explain why neuropsychiatric problems are real and how they can result from a combination of brain injury to certain parts of the brain and other medical and environmental factors. Unfortunately, a stigma still surrounds neuropsychiatric problems, stemming from the mistaken belief that they are not as "real" as physical symptoms. But these problems are as real as physical problems. Just as people with sensory problems (like blindness) or motor deficits (like paralysis) have damage to certain brain circuits, people with neuropsychiatric problems may have damage to brain circuits that modulate their mood, control their impulses, manage their memories, and allow them to act and think in socially appropriate ways.

We don't want to describe only the problems of brain injury. We also want to focus on the brain's ability to heal. We discuss the concept of neural plasticity—that is, the brain's ability to change and compensate for injury. We also discuss various ways that the brain's natural ability to heal can be augmented, ranging from behavioral techniques to brain stimulation techniques to meditation.

This book is divided into a number of parts. In the first part, we discuss how the brain works. In the second part, we discuss in detail neural plasticity and its relevance after brain injury. We then devote much of the rest of the chapters to explaining the major emotional, behavioral, and cognitive issues that can arise after brain injury. In these chapters, we present typical case studies and discuss treatments to help patients and their families. We summarize the discussion by providing tips and tools the person with brain injury and their caregiver can use. We conclude each chapter by providing take-home points and a simple exercise the person with brain injury can do. The chapters offer specific behavioral methods to help manage problems following brain injury and help leverage neural plasticity to heal. We cite cases describing people with whom we have worked, but to maintain privacy and for the purpose of confidentiality, we have made changes to all identifiable information.

Additionally, we devote a few chapters to specific methods that may help the brain to heal. We discuss the latest technologies in brain stimulation, and we also discuss ancient knowledge that has stood the test of time and has increasing support, such as yoga and meditation. We hope this book brings help and hope to persons with brain injury and their families as they embark on a journey of recovery of the traumatized brain.

A note of caution: This book should not and cannot be used for self-treatment of brain injury. The services of a medical professional are essential for appropriate treatment. Furthermore, no person should take a prescription medication unless a licensed physician has specifically prescribed it for them after proper medical evaluation. No person should take a medication, adjust the dose of a medication, or stop taking a medication without first consulting their physician. Any person taking a prescription medication should be supervised and monitored by a physician for the duration of the prescription.

Part I

Brain Structure
and Function

In this part, we focus on brain structure and function. It can be useful to understand how the brain operates so that the effects of damage to the brain make more sense. After all, to understand dysfunction, it is helpful to understand normal function. We try to minimize extraneous detail and excessive technicality, but you can certainly skip this section if you wish. You may want to use this section as a reference to come back to as needed.

In chapter 1, we look at the brain at a cellular level. We introduce a number of terms necessary to communicate about the brain. This may be helpful to readers who wish to understand the medical terminology used by doctors (see also the glossary near the end of the book).

In chapter 2, we look at the brain at a structural level, that is, at different parts of the brain. We focus in this chapter, as we do throughout, on parts of the brain that are involved with mood, behavior, and cognitive processing.

In chapter 3, we build on the first two chapters and make the transition from normal function to dysfunction, from normality to pathology. We discuss different types of brain injury and their impact on different aspects of the brain.

Finally, in chapter 4, we discuss how the brain can recover; we

explain that the brain is always dynamic, always learning, always malleable—characteristics that are the basis of the behavioral advice we
offer later in the book in discussing how to improve specific symptoms after brain injury.

Chapter 1

Inner Workings

The brain is a part of the body's complex nervous system, whose differ-ent parts are described in figure 1.1. Main functions of the nervous system include collecting information from the five sensory organs (eyes, ears, skin, nose, and tongue), processing this information, and reacting appropriately, using internal goals and emotions to guide action.

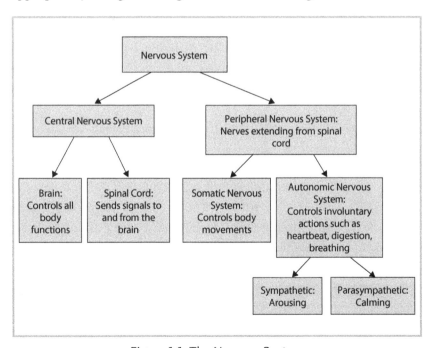

Figure 1.1. The Nervous System

The brain is a three-pound mass of gelatinous material that allows us to be who we are. It is amazing that this critical seat of our body's operation weighs so little and is the consistency of really overcooked cauliflower. Despite its humble size, it is where we humans develop and store our unique personalities, emotions, and dreams for the future. It contains our sense of our unique self. It allows us to remember, speak, think, plan, and move. The brain has a privileged position in our body: it is in many ways the conductor, the maestro, coordinating the orchestra of the body. Through its connections to the nerves and the spinal cord, the brain controls the beating of our heart, the digestion in our gastrointestinal tract, the workings of our lungs. Even more fundamentally, the brain allows us to be awake, conscious, and aware of our surroundings.

The brain's fundamental unit of operation is the brain cell, called a neuron, whose function and connections are described in figure 1.2 and table 1.1. There are a *lot* of neurons in the human brain, something on the order of 86 billion.

In addition to neurons, the brain includes other cells, called glial cells. We used to think that glial cells were there only to support neurons, but it may be that glial cells do more than that—they may also, like neurons, contribute to the brain's ability to deliver and send messages (and may even outnumber neurons), thus adding to the brain's computing power.

Neurons are electrochemical units, meaning that they require both electric current and chemicals to function. The electrical process depends on the concentration of charged atoms (known as ions) like sodium, potassium, chloride, and calcium. Differing concentrations of these particles inside and outside the neuron create voltage differences across the neuron membrane (the outer "skin" of the cell). At baseline, neurons have a net negative internal charge. When positive ions such as sodium or potassium enter the neuron, the electrical charge inside the cell becomes less negative. When this charge becomes significantly less negative, the neuron fires, meaning that electrical current flows across the neuron and down an axon (see table 1.1 for a definition of terms). When the electrical current reaches the end of the axon, a group of

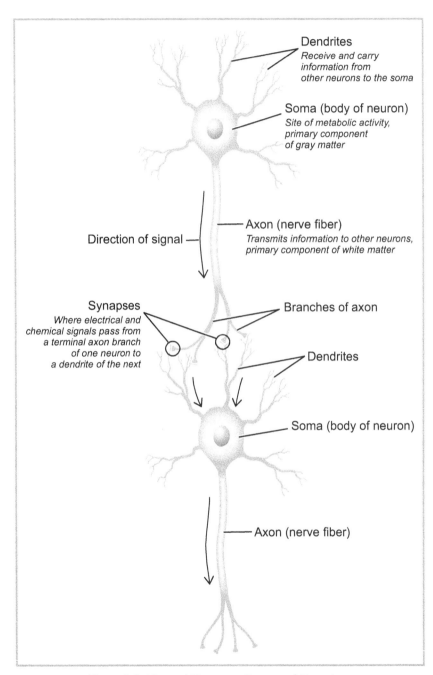

Dendrites
*Receive and carry
information from
other neurons to the soma*

Soma (body of neuron)
*Site of metabolic activity,
primary component
of gray matter*

Axon (nerve fiber)
*Transmits information to other neurons,
primary component of white matter*

Direction of signal

Synapses
*Where electrical and
chemical signals pass from
a terminal axon branch
of one neuron to
a dendrite of the next*

Branches of axon

Dendrites

Soma (body of neuron)

Axon (nerve fiber)

Figure 1.2. Normal Neurons: Parts and Functions

TABLE 1.1. PARTS AND FUNCTIONS OF A NEURON

Part	Description	Function
Soma	Cell body	Powerhouse of the neuron; maintains its functioning
Axon	Cylindrical structure emanating from the cell body	Carries messages from the cell body to other neurons
Dendrite	Branch from the cell body	Receives messages from other neurons
Synapse	Space between any two neurons	Enables communication by passing electrical and chemical signals from one neuron to another

chemicals called neurotransmitters flow into the synapse. These neu-rotransmitters include chemicals like serotonin, norepinephrine, dopa-mine, glutamate, and gamma-aminobutyric acid (GABA). Once the neurotransmitters are released, they lock onto receptors on the next neuron. This coupling then changes the voltage of that neuron, making it, in turn, more or less likely to fire. This is a simplistic explanation of what happens in the brain: in reality, each neuron has input from multiple other neurons at its dendrites, perhaps up to 10,000 at the same time. Whether a certain neuron fires or not, whether it excites or inhibits the next neuron, is based on complex dynamics.

Neurons group together into pathways, or circuits, that carry out certain functions. For example, one circuit, called the corticospinal tract, allows us to move our body. The corticospinal tract begins in the motor cortex in the brain, travels through the brainstem into the spinal cord, and then through peripheral nerves to the muscles. This circuit thus includes a large number of neurons, all communicating and coor-dinating with one another by means of electricity and chemicals. The corticospinal tract is categorized as a motor circuit.

Sensory circuits allow us to gather information from the environment. Separate circuits exist for pain and temperature, light touch and vibration, vision, hearing, smell, taste, and more. Motor circuits help us act. Coordination circuits control how we orchestrate our movements, allowing us to move fluidly.

In addition to the motor, sensory, and coordination circuits, the brain has a number of more complex pathways called higher-order circuits. These circuits regulate our mood, thinking, memory, impulse control, and personality, among other things. They control what we think of as "selves," the qualities that make us human, that make us who we are. Underlying the motor, sensory, and coordination circuits are circuits that control consciousness itself, the ability to be awake, alert, and sentient.

The idea that these higher-order circuits are responsible for creating who we are is a fundamental but controversial concept. We may hesitate at some level to believe that there are circuits in the brain that make up our personality, our motivations, our intentions—the qualities that make us "us." A fundamental tenet of modern neuroscience (the scientific study of the nervous system) is that damage to these higher-order circuits results in neuropsychiatric symptoms such as depression, anxiety, memory loss, and abnormal behavior. Brain injury can damage these very circuits, affecting those who suffer from brain injury in fundamental ways.

We like to believe that we are more than just the sum of our circuits and that we have a sense of control over our destinies. We all believe that we have intention and can come up with a plan and then execute that plan. Simplistically stated, we can think of our intentions and plans as software programs. However, to make the best use of the software, the hardware or the infrastructure of the brain, particularly higher-order circuitry, must be intact. Without that intact infrastructure, our intentions and plans cannot be carried out the way we want them to. We may have the most sophisticated software programs, but if we are running them on a damaged computer, we cannot take advantage of the software. Similarly, if the hardware of the brain is not intact, we cannot control our emotions, our plans, our dreams.

Clearly, then, to understand the software of our behavior, we have to understand the hardware that is the brain. By focusing on the brain and its circuitry, we are not minimizing the human condition. We do agree that our thinking, emotions, and behavior are dependent on both nature and nurture; the development of our brain circuitry is based on genes and the environment with which we interact.

Our brain is changing all the time, as we deal with our environment, as we react to new information. Our brain has to be dynamic or we would not do very well in a constantly changing world. Humans have evolved to a point where we dominate other species largely because our brains are so dynamic and adaptable. This dynamism is also reflected in our brain circuitry.

All the richness and complexity of our mental lives, our moods, our behaviors, our thinking and memory are based on the interaction of brain circuits laid down as our brains developed as babies and on changes to these circuits as we accumulated environmental experiences. Some research also suggests that chronic stress and adverse experiences during childhood can change the brain. In other words, we are not who we are only because our brains were fated to develop in a certain way, and we are not who we are only because of the environments in which we find ourselves. We are who we are because of a combination of both—of nature and nurture.

This notion is similar to current thinking about our genetic code. Our DNA does not doom us inevitably to develop certain illnesses. Of course, our genetic code does predispose us to particular illnesses because it reflects contributions from our genetic predecessors. However, environmental factors, both good and bad, can affect how these genes are expressed. By changing our behavior—exercising, eating certain foods, and perhaps taking certain medications as prescribed—we may be able to change how our genes are expressed. There is even emerging evidence that the bacteria and viruses we carry in our bodies (called the microbiome) can affect how our genes are expressed. Ongoing animal research is studying how products released by these microbiomes can affect the brain and how certain brain conditions can impact the gut. The butterflies we experience in our stomach when we are stressed may be an example of the gut-brain connection.

We can, in some ways, then, change our fate, at least to some degree. Nevertheless, we should be aware of the genetic sequences we are born with because they are the basis of what may happen to us in the future. Similarly, we should understand our brain circuits, because they are the basis of how we are who we are.

In chapter 2, we look at the brain's structures in greater detail and discuss what they do. You may skip the next chapter if you feel that the information there is too technical or not relevant at the moment; you can always return to it later. We do hope, though, that you will join us as we explore the structures of the brain, which, in many ways, make us who we are, and let us think, feel, dream, remember, and plan.

TAKE-HOME POINTS

The brain is a part of a complex body system called the nervous system.

The brain allows us to be who we are. It allows us to remember, speak, think, plan, and move; it allows us to have our unique personalities, our emotions, and our dreams for the future.

Our thinking, emotions, and behavior are dependent on both nature and nurture, the genes we have, and the environment we interact with.

Chapter 2

Structure

In chapter 1 we introduced a number of terms and focused on the brain at a cellular and neuronal level. In this chapter, we explore the structure of the brain—its parts and how they work together. We discuss the major components of the brain, including the cerebral cortex, the cerebellum, the basal ganglia, the thalamus, the hypothalamus, and the brainstem.

The brain consists of two types of tissue: white matter and gray matter. White matter consists of long strands of axons, called axon tracts, which connect the different parts of the brain. White matter carries the signals or messages to different parts of the brain. A layer of fatty tissue, called myelin, which protects the axons and helps in signal transmission, covers the axons. The fat in myelin appears white, hence the name *white matter*.

Gray matter contains the neurons, as well as other supporting cells, including glial cells. Within the gray matter, neurons connect and form synapses. Gray matter contains only cells and small blood vessels and lacks white myelin.

Although the various regions of the brain connect and work together, structurally the brain is divided into distinct areas, each of which has its unique function. The major regions of the brain are illustrated in figures 2.1a and 2.1b.

The brainstem, located in the back of the brain, connects with the spinal cord. It is composed of the midbrain, pons, and medulla, and it

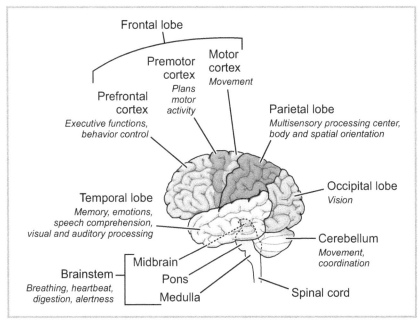

Figure 2.1a. Side View of the Brain

is critical to life. Groups of cells distributed throughout the brainstem compose a network called the reticular activating system (RAS). The RAS allows us to be conscious, alert, and aware. Damage to the RAS results in unconsciousness.

The lowest section of the brainstem, the medulla, controls critical moment-to-moment automatic functions like breathing and heartbeat. The pons portion of the brainstem plays a role in generating dreams during sleep. The midbrain is important for movement and pain processing. Axon tracts carrying sensory and motor information travel through the brainstem to and from the spinal cord, so damage to the brainstem can lead to paralysis or a devastating condition called locked-in syndrome, in which the person is conscious and aware but is unable to move any portion of the body except the eyes. Because cognitive activities like thinking and memory are not housed in the brainstem, damage to the brainstem does not typically affect these higher-order functions.

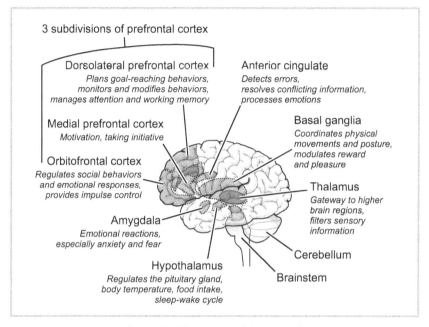

Figure 2.1b. Medial (Deep Inside) View of the Brain

Sitting above the brainstem is the thalamus. As the relay system of sensory information, the thalamus is a critical part of the brain's interconnected architecture. It receives input from the environment (through vision, hearing, touch), processes it, and then sends it to the rest of the brain. The thalamus filters out "unnecessary" sensory stimuli so that the rest of the brain is not overwhelmed with information. It is involved in thought, and therefore people who have damage to the thalamus can be confused and disoriented. The thalamus is also critical to our ability to pay attention, and in particular it plays a role in spatial attention. It is also involved in processing pain.

Below the thalamus lies the hypothalamus. This portion of the brain is involved in expressing rage, appetite, and sexual behaviors. The hypothalamus controls the nearby pituitary gland, the so-called master gland of the body, which secretes chemicals called hormones, such as growth hormone and thyroid-stimulating hormone, affecting the actions of many body organs.

The cerebellum, at the back of the brain near the brainstem, helps with movement, particularly the ability to coordinate balance. People who have damage to the cerebellum have trouble walking in a straight line. Alcohol can impair the cerebellum, which is why police sobriety tests include walking heel-to-toe and touching the finger to the nose in a smooth, direct fashion. Yet the cerebellum's role is not limited to movement; it may also be involved with the coordination and fluidity of both thought and speech.

Deep within the brain, near the center and bordering the thalamus, lie two sets of structures, called the basal ganglia, that are also involved with movement. The basal ganglia are composed of four distinct groups of cells, called nuclei. The four nuclei are the putamen, the caudate, the subthalamic nucleus, and the globus pallidus. Within each set of basal ganglia on either side of the brain, these nuclei form circuits that smooth out our movements. Parkinson's disease and other movement disorders affect this area of the brain. Damage to the basal ganglia can result in tremor and walking difficulties. The basal ganglia also have important roles in cognition, and several circuits connect the basal ganglia to the frontal lobes of the brain. Part of the basal ganglia (the ventral striatum and, more specifically, the nucleus accumbens) is important for our sense of pleasure and reward. In people with brain injury, dysfunction of this circuit can lead to excessive need for a quick reward despite the potential that the behavior could be risky, or the other extreme, where nothing is rewarding

The cerebral cortex is the outer covering of the brain, consisting of many folds and ridges. The cortex is highly developed in humans, and this sophistication is believed to be one critical factor that differentiates humans from other animals. The cortex is composed of four divisions called lobes—the frontal lobe, temporal lobe, parietal lobe, and occipital lobe. There is a duplicate set of lobes on each side of the brain.

The frontal lobe plays an important part in higher-order cognitive activities like thinking, planning, goal setting, organizing thoughts, abstracting, and conceptualizing. It also is important in organizing movements. The frontal lobe consists of the motor cortex, the premotor cortex, and the prefrontal cortex. As their names suggest, the motor cortex and premotor cortex are associated with movement. The frontal lobe, particularly the prefrontal cortex, is often known as the chief executive officer of the brain because of its role in coordinating other brain regions.

The prefrontal cortex itself has three regions: the ventral prefrontal cortex (with the orbitofrontal cortex as the main component), the dorsolateral prefrontal cortex, and the medial prefrontal cortex. The prefrontal cortex is involved in cognitive activity. Damage or dysfunction of the orbitofrontal cortex, which can occur with brain injury (particularly traumatic brain injury), can lead to significant personality changes—for example, not caring about social conventions. Individuals with damage to this part of the brain become focused on their own wants, needs, and desires and as a result, present as self-centered. Excessive activity in the orbitofrontal cortex can cause repetitive thoughts and behaviors, as happens in obsessive-compulsive disorder. The dorsolateral prefrontal cortex is mainly associated with cognitive functioning, specifically executive functions such as planning, organizing, abstract reasoning, and inhibition, and it contributes to cognitive flexibility and working memory. In addition, in its connections with other regions of the brain, the dorsolateral prefrontal cortex also contributes to mood changes such as depression. The dorsolateral prefrontal cortex is frequently damaged in brain injury, contributing to problems with cognitive activity and mood changes.

The temporal lobes house circuits involved in processing visual and auditory information. Damage to the temporal lobes can lead to visual problems, trouble with hearing, and even auditory hallucinations (as in schizophrenia). In the inside (or medial) part of the temporal lobe, one circuit is involved in short-term memory storage and processing. The medial temporal lobe contains the hippocampus, a crucial structure in memory formation. Alzheimer's disease is associated with damage to the hippocampus. Similarly, people with brain injury who have damage to the temporal lobe can have problems remembering newly learned information.

Deeper inside the brain, near the temporal lobe, is a circuit historically called the limbic system, which regulates our emotions. The limbic system includes the amygdala, the mammillary body, and the cingulate gyrus, among other structures. Research indicates that excess activity in parts of the limbic system, particularly in the amygdala, is related to high levels of anxiety.

The front part of the cingulate gyrus, the anterior cingulate, seems to be crucial for cognitive functions (for example, detecting errors and resolving conflicts), motivation, emotional processing, and pain. This region may also have a role in the development of anxiety and depressive symptoms. Research suggests that deep-brain stimulation of a particular region of the anterior cingulate may be helpful in treating depressive symptoms.

The occipital lobes are important for vision, and damage to them can lead to blindness. Different parts of each of the occipital lobes allow us to recognize shape, visual movement, and color. Visual information, once processed in the occipital lobes, is sent on to the temporal lobes for further analysis; the temporal lobe areas that connect to the occipital lobes help us identify faces and integrate the various attributes of a given object (movement with shape, for example).

In this chapter we have provided a brief overview of the major parts of the brain. It is important to note, though, that even though these parts of the brain are critical for specific activities, the interconnectedness of the brain makes its function highly complex. Damage to any one area of the brain can set off a string of repercussions to physical, emotional, and cognitive health. Indeed, another way to think about the brain is to think less in terms of specific areas, and more in terms of circuits or networks. For example, brain functioning can be thought of as the interaction of at least 15 circuits. The cognitive control network (also known as the central executive network), the salience network, and the default mode network are particularly important for neuropsychiatric symptoms.

The predominant brain regions of the cognitive control network include the dorsolateral prefrontal cortex and the posterior parietal cortex. As the name suggests, this network focuses on cognitive tasks. The default mode network includes the medial prefrontal cortex, medial temporal lobe, posterior cingulate cortex, and parts of the medial parietal lobe. It is activated by inner thought, when there is no particular external task that the brain has to do. It is thought to be important for multiple functions, including memory. Alzheimer's disease may in fact start in the default mode network. The salience network is important to recognize and process salient objects (*salience* is from a root word that suggests jumping out; something salient is important and "jumps out" at someone). Predominant brain regions of the salience network include the anterior insula and parts of the anterior cingulate cortex. The salience network may be important in having brain activity switch between the default mode network (inner thought) to the cognitive control network (an external task). As an example, if a person is crossing a busy street and then suddenly a bus turns the corner and appears on that street, the salience network recognizes a salient object (a bus coming at the person) and gets the brain to switch from inner thought to being more task oriented (getting out of the way of the bus).

The most comprehensive and accurate way to think about brain structure is to think about critical nodes (brain regions) in multiple networks. Some of the critical nodes can be used in multiple roles and in multiple networks. This is similar to a flight network in which certain critical hubs (or nodes) can be used in multiple different flight patterns. Ultimately, the system is designed to be resilient; if one airport has to close for some reason, other airports can take those flights to some extent. Similarly, the brain has a modular structure (certain important regions), but also has a mosaic structure (networks that include these nodes that are malleable and dynamic, providing greater resilience).

TAKE-HOME POINTS

The brain is a uniquely organized structure that includes different regions (also called lobes) with distinct functions.

The different regions are also intricately connected with each other in an organized manner, forming circuits or networks.

Damage to one part of the brain by any mechanism (such as trauma, stroke, or tumor) can cause damage or dysfunction not only to that region, but also to other areas to which the component is connected.

Chapter 3

Types of
Brain Injury

Brain injury can damage different parts of the brain in many ways. Broadly speaking, brain damage can be congenital or acquired. Congenital brain injury is damage that occurs before birth, at birth, or just after birth. Acquired brain injury (figure 3.1) is damage that occurs well after birth, with a clear cause of the injury. In other words, it is unrelated to birth events and is not hereditary or congenital. This book focuses only on acquired brain injuries.

Depending on the severity of injury, the consequences of brain damage range from absence of symptoms to mild to severe symptoms and sometimes even death. The severity of symptoms is usually proportional to the severity and type of brain injury. In this chapter, we describe the most common causes of brain injury and how those injuries affect brain tissue. Although the medical words and phrases we introduce here might be overwhelming, it is important to be familiar with them because you may hear them from your doctor. Our aim is to help you understand the bewildering terminology of brain injury and give you a better sense of how brain injuries can happen. Also, it is important to note that independent of the cause of injury or symptoms that emerge, treatment should be multipronged, taking into consideration the person's coping skills, medications, and lifestyle modification. We stress the multipronged approach of management throughout this book.

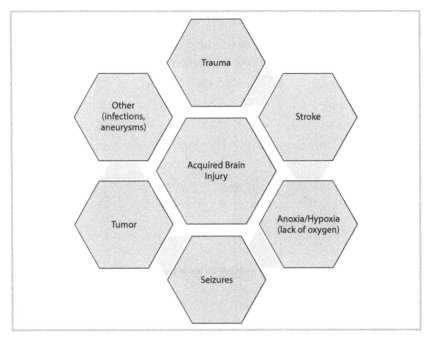

Figure 3.1. Common Causes of Acquired Brain Injury

Traumatic Brain Injury

The most common causes of traumatic brain injury, or TBI, include impact injury, penetrating injury, injury from inertial forces, and blast injury.

An impact injury occurs when the head makes sudden, forceful contact with some object: the brain accelerates, and then abruptly stops. An example of this is a fall: when a person falls, the brain accelerates as gravity pulls the body down, then suddenly stops when the head hits the ground.

In a penetrating injury, an object penetrates the brain. An example is a bullet that passes through the skull into the brain. The trajectory (path) and speed of the bullet directly damage the brain. Changes in air pressure caused by the traveling bullet can also damage brain tissue. Because they cause direct damage to the brain tissue, penetrating injuries can lead to tissue death and irritation of the brain, which can cause seizures.

Injury from inertial forces (also known as acceleration and deceleration injury) results when the brain moves within the skull, but without head impact. An example of this is a car accident in which the head jerks suddenly when the car is hit by another vehicle, but the head does not hit the windshield.

Finally, there is blast injury, which most frequently occurs in the context of war or a bomb explosion. Shock waves from explosions are believed to be the cause of brain damage because of the sudden change in pressure brought on by the exploding device. Blast injuries are now more prevalent in American military personnel due to the recent wars in the Middle East and Afghanistan.

Types of Brain Damage from Traumatic Brain Injury

Each form of TBI causes distinct types of damage. Similarly, each type of damage has its own unique consequences. Common types of brain damage are described in table 3.1.

Contusion

Contusion, or bruising of the brain, commonly occurs in impact injuries. The force of the impact "throws" the brain into the skull, damaging the soft tissue. For example, the front of the head hitting a solid object can cause a contusion in the frontal lobes. This impact is called a coup injury. Coup injuries are often followed immediately by a contrecoup injury, when the impact of the object jostles the brain within the skull, which damages the opposite area of the brain.

Among the contributors to contusions after a direct hit to the brain are bony areas and ridges on the interior of the skull overlying the frontal and temporal lobes. These irregular surfaces protrude into the skull cavity, making the frontal and temporal lobes more vulnerable to injury. As discussed elsewhere in this book, damage to the frontal and temporal lobes can cause significant mood, behavioral, and cognitive changes. Damage to these areas may not be immediately obvious to family and friends because the person may be able to move and talk normally, but

TABLE 3.1. TYPES OF BRAIN DAMAGE

Type of damage	Description
Contusion	Bruising of the brain
Skull	Break in the bone covering the brain
Epidural	Collection of blood between the skull and a thin outer covering of the brain called the dura mater
Subdural	Collection of blood between the outermost layer covering the brain (dura mater) and the middle layer covering the brain (arachnoid membrane)
Subarachnoid	Collection of blood in the subarachnoid space— between the arachnoid membrane and the innermost layer covering the brain (pia mater)
Intracerebral	Bleeding within the brain
Increased	Any collection of blood inside the brain or outside that causes an increase in pressure inside the brain and cerebrospinal fluid
Anoxic	Complete lack of oxygen or decreased oxygen to the brain
Diffuse	Injury to the white matter fibers of the brain

there can be significant changes in personality—that is, a meaningful change from who the person was before the injury.

Skull Fracture

A particularly forceful blow to the head can fracture the skull. Fractures can be penetrating, such as when a fractured bony chip penetrates into the brain, or non-penetrating, when there is no penetration of bony fragments into the brain. Penetrating skull fractures are more likely than other traumas to cause bleeding within the brain. People who sustain a skull fracture may be more likely to develop seizures. The phrase "brain laceration" describes brain tissue that is physically cut or torn, either by the pushed-in bone fragment from a skull fracture or by a foreign object such as a bullet or bullet fragment from a gunshot wound.

Bleeding in the Brain

The medical term for bleeding within the brain is *intracranial hemorrhage*. There are two types of intracranial hemorrhage: those between the brain and the skull (called epidural hemorrhages, subdural hemorrhages, or subarachnoid hemorrhages, based on their location) and those within the brain itself (called intracerebral hemorrhage), all described in table 3.1. The words hematoma and hemorrhage are easily confused. Hemorrhage means active bleeding, whereas hematoma means clotted blood or a collection of blood outside a blood vessel (for example, an artery, a vein, or capillaries) into a tissue space such as brain tissue or joint. Hematomas can be small or large. Symptoms from a hematoma depend on its size and whether it is exerting pressure on nearby tissue.

An epidural hematoma is a collection of blood right below the skull, between the skull and a thin outer covering of the brain called the dura mater. Epidural hematomas usually occur in the temporal areas, and their cause is often injury to the side of the head. The majority occur because of damage to the meningeal arteries, but a small proportion can also be due to damage to veins. Because the blood in all arteries is under higher pressure than blood in veins, leaking blood can quickly accumulate and injure the brain. Epidural hematomas cause brain damage because the pool of leaking blood can press down on the adjacent brain, indenting and flattening it. The result is lack of oxygen (called anoxic injury) in the tissue that is being compressed. Epidural hematomas are almost always medical emergencies.

A subdural hematoma is also a collection of blood between the brain and the skull, but below the dura mater membrane. Subdural hematomas are closer to the brain than epidural hematomas, but they are still outside the brain. Subdural hematomas tend to arise from tears in veins as opposed to arteries, so they accumulate more slowly than epidural hematomas, because veins are under less pressure than arteries. Subdural hematomas develop most often in older adults, whose veins are more fragile and have stretched because of underlying brain atrophy (shrinkage). Older adults and people who abuse alcohol are particularly prone to subdural hematomas—and sometimes repeated subdural hematomas—because they are more likely to fall or bump their head. The blood in a subdural hematoma can collect slowly, so the person with this type of injury may not be immediately aware of the injury. Subdural hematomas may resolve spontaneously or may require surgery.

A subarachnoid hemorrhage is a collection of blood even closer to the brain than a subdural hematoma, but still outside the brain. Subarachnoid hemorrhages develop below the arachnoid mater—yet another membrane covering the brain—and beneath the dura mater. They can occur as a result of trauma, ruptured cerebral aneurysm (which is a ballooning of an artery in the brain), or ruptured arteriovenous malformation (which is an abnormal connection between the blood vessels). Subarachnoid hemorrhages are also considered life-threatening.

An intracerebral hemorrhage is bleeding within the brain. This injury commonly occurs in the frontal and temporal lobes. Severe impact injury can cause both contusions on the brain surface and bleeding within the brain. Impacts of great force, such as car accidents, are common causes of intracerebral hemorrhages. Because blood is irritating to the brain, intracerebral hemorrhage can cause seizures.

Pressure on the Brain

Any form of bleeding either outside or within the brain can increase the pressure in the brain tissue and cerebrospinal fluid (fluid surrounding the brain and spinal cord). In an epidural hematoma, blood can quickly expand and collect, pressing on the brain with increasing force. Such increased pressure can become a serious problem because the skull does not allow the brain to expand from the swelling. Additional pressure on the brain, however, forces the brain to move somewhere. Elevated pressure can push it into the opening at the bottom of the skull, a hole through which the spine connects to the brain. The diameter of this hole is much smaller than the brain, so any part of the brain driven into this hole is essentially strangled, resulting in a condition called herniation. Herniation of this type can lead to death, because it affects the lower part of the brain, which controls breathing.

Oxygen Deprivation

As noted above, the consequences of TBI include not only direct damage to brain tissue, but also bleeding in the brain, which can have consequences beyond just increased pressure; bleeding can endanger the brain's oxygen supply. Red blood cells in the bloodstream carry oxygen molecules, so a bleeding blood vessel reduces the oxygen supply to the brain. The result is called an anoxic (absence of oxygen) or hypoxic (decreased oxygen) injury. Anoxic/hypoxic injury can also lead to inflammation, which in turn can lead to the death of brain cells.

There are many other causes of anoxic/hypoxic brain damage. Examples include stroke, strangulation (either related to domestic violence or suicide attempt by hanging), near drowning, drug overdose with narcotics (opiates, heroin) or sedatives/tranquilizers (benzodiazepines).

Damage to Neurons

Trauma to the brain can cause injury to the neurons and also injury to the axons, all of which can interfere with normal brain functioning. (Common types of brain cell injuries resulting from a TBI are shown in figure 3.2.) Axons are connecting fibers between neurons that form the white matter tissue of the brain. The back-and-forth movement of the soft brain within the bony skull during trauma can stretch and tear the axons, a condition known as diffuse axonal injury (DAI). These TBIs occur in inertial injuries, particularly those occurring in car accidents in which the head is not hit but the brain moves within the skull. If severe enough, DAI can lead to coma and death—if the axons stretch

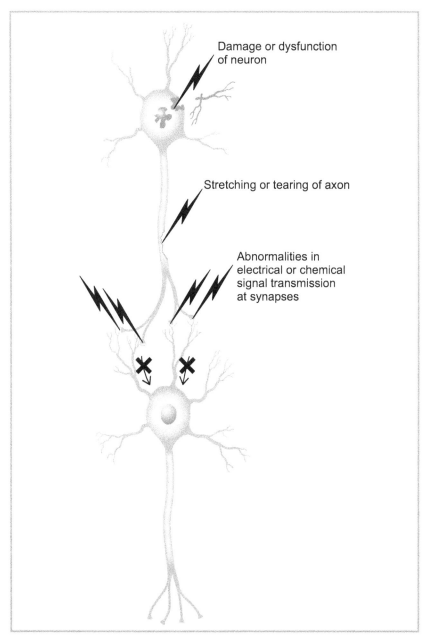

Damage or dysfunction of neuron

Stretching or tearing of axon

Abnormalities in electrical or chemical signal transmission at synapses

Figure 3.2. Types of Injuries to Neurons That Can Result from Traumatic Brain Injuries

so hard or so far that they snap and detach from the neuron. Mild TBIs or concussions can result from diffuse axonal injuries, which may be temporary or permanent depending on the number and frequency of injuries. DAI is not detected by conventional brain imaging studies, such as computerized tomography (CT). A more sophisticated form of magnetic resonance imaging called diffusion tensor imaging (DTI) is better than CT or standard MRI (magnetic resonance imaging) at detecting axonal injuries. DTI and other new scanning techniques are mainly research tools at present, but they may be used in the future to evaluate people for DAI.

Stroke

Strokes are another type of brain injury. Most strokes are ischemic, meaning that they are due to a blood clot in the brain. Just like heart attacks are due to a clot in the coronary arteries, most strokes are due to clots in vessels in the brain. Strokes are brain attacks. They can also occur because of bleeding in the brain (these are called hemorrhagic strokes), as noted previously.

Strokes can be obvious, leading to paralysis or speaking difficulties (aphasias). However, they can occur in areas of the brain that are not detected by a neurological exam but that can affect mood, behavior, and memory. One of the critical principles of our understanding of the brain is that the actual cause of damage may not be as important as the locales of the brain that are affected and the circuits that may be damaged.

Brain Tumor

Brain tumors are unfortunately not uncommon. In adults, often diagnosis is made after a seizure in a person with no history of seizure. This is because brain tumors tend to irritate the surrounding brain tissue, leading to increased neuronal activity and eventually seizures. Sometimes the brain tumor is large enough that it causes swelling, which can lead to headaches and symptoms from distant parts of the brain affected by the swelling.

There are many ways to classify tumors based on pathology or based on genetic markers. Another method is to divide brain tumors into primary or metastatic types.

Primary brain tumors arise from the brain directly, typically from glial cells, which include astrocytes and oligodendrocytes. Glial cells were traditionally thought to provide metabolic and structural support to neurons, but it is becoming more evident that glial cells themselves are important in the computational functions of the brain. Astrocytes in particular may be important in regulating neurotransmitter levels in synapses. Oligodendrocytes are important in allowing neuronal signals to be transmitted quickly throughout the brain.

Primary brain tumors can be classified as low-grade or high-grade tumors. Low-grade tumors are classified as WHO (World Health Organization) Grade I or II tumors. Grade III and IV tumors are considered high-grade. These tumors have worse outcomes, particularly Grade IV tumors, which are also known as GBMs (glioblastoma multiforme). There can be a wide variation in average time to death based on the grade of the tumor (months to many years). The genetic markers of the tumor can also affect survivability, with better survivability with some markers (*IDH1*, *IDH2*, *1p19q*, and *MGMT* mutations), and worse survivability with other markers (such as *TERT* mutations). Metastatic brain tumors spread to the brain from other organs. For example, prostate or breast cancer may spread to the brain. The consequences of metastatic brain tumors are similar to other forms of brain injury, with damage to circuits determining the symptoms.

Unfortunately, treatment for brain tumors, such as surgery and radiation, can themselves cause a brain injury. Surgery is inherently violent and relatively nonspecific, resecting the tumor but also disrupting normal brain matter and pathways. Radiation targets a tumor, but it can also cause damage to white matter pathways that connect the brain, damage that can lead to slowed thinking and attention and memory problems. Even though medications used to treat cancer (chemotherapy) can be helpful, side effects of the medications can be associated with memory problems and mental fogginess. Some people call this condition chemo brain. We are still not clear about the mechanisms causing chemo brain, but it is important to remember that there may be many other factors causing the symptoms, such as stress, poor sleep, and inadequate nutrition.

Epilepsy

Epilepsy can cause brain injury due to repeated uncontrolled seizures, which can lead to hypoxia, and hypoxia leads to brain injury, as we have discussed. Seizures can be focal (or partial) or be generalized.

Simple partial seizures do not include any changes in awareness; rather, depending on what circuit is affected, there can be sensory, motor, mood, or behavioral symptoms. There can be numbness in a certain part of the body, temporary weakness of a limb, a sudden change in mood, or difficulty speaking.

Generalized seizures can affect both sides of the brain and affect awareness. The most well-known type of a generalized seizure is a generalized tonic-clonic seizure. With this seizure, there is loss of awareness (consciousness), increased muscle contractions, and rhythmic shaking. If the seizure lasts more than five minutes, it is considered a medical emergency (called status epilepticus) due to risk of damage to the brain because of lack of oxygen.

Other Types of Brain Injury

Dementias (such as Alzheimer's disease) are neurodegenerative diseases where there is not a static brain injury (like the other brain injuries we have considered so far); rather, there is ongoing injury to the brain, leading to an often-unrelenting progressive worsening of symptoms. We focus on static brain injuries in this book, so we will not discuss dementias much. But, as with other forms of brain injury, dementias damage brain circuits, leading to predictable mood, behavioral, and cognitive symptoms.

Multiple sclerosis can also be considered a form of brain injury. Multiple sclerosis is due to an autoimmune process whereby the body attacks the brain, with the immune system attacking the nervous system. This damage tends to occur mostly in the white matter fibers that connect the brain, leading classically to slowed thinking (as with radiation). Mood changes can also occur, which can lead to significant depression. The most common form of multiple sclerosis is the relapsing-remitting type, which entails flares of worsening autoimmune attacks with periods of relative sparing of attacks. These flares can be assessed with MRIs, as they show new white matter lesions. Over time, some people can convert from the relapsing-remitting type to the secondary progressive type, which worsens or progresses in a continuous manner. There is also a primary progressive type of multiple sclerosis, where the disease is progressive from the onset.

In this chapter, we have reviewed the major types and mechanics of traumatic brain injury, bleeding within and outside of the brain, seizures, swelling, and brain injury due to stroke, seizures, and multiple sclerosis. Brain bleeds are life-threatening conditions requiring immediate medical care. Consult with a medical professional at the first sign of new or abnormal symptoms after brain injury, such as headache, dizziness, confusion, disorientation, or fogginess. Other common symptoms of brain injuries are loss of consciousness, sudden severe headache, seizures, vomiting, weakness in the arms or legs, difficulty speaking, or sudden changes in vision.

In chapter 4 we build upon the knowledge we have gained and discuss how the brain can recover from the various types of injuries we discussed. We focus on the notion of brain plasticity—the dynamic nature of the brain. The brain is able to change, and indeed, it is changing all the time as it processes and learns new information. We discuss how this notion is relevant to recovery from brain injury.

TAKE-HOME POINTS

There are many causes of acquired brain injury. Examples include trauma, stroke, and tumor.

Damage to the brain can be secondary to one or more factors: bleeding, swelling of the brain, inflammation, deprivation of oxygen, damage to neurons or axons.

Consult with a medical professional at the first sign of new or abnormal symptoms after a brain injury.

Older adults are more vulnerable to a blow/injury than they might have been in their youth because of age-related changes in the brain. Any observed or reported hit to the head or fall of an older adult should be checked out.

Chapter 4

Influences on Recovery after Brain Injury

On a foggy October morning, Wilson, a 67-year-old man, was involved in a multivehicle crash on a country road. He was driving the fourth of five vehicles in the accident chain. The fifth car plowed into the back of Wilson's car at about 50 miles per hour, driving his car into and under the car in front of him. Wilson sustained cuts and bruises to his face. He apparently never lost consciousness, but the emergency medical services team found him dazed and disoriented at the scene of the accident, so they transported him to the local emergency department for evaluation. The results of a computerized tomography (CT) scan of his head and neck were normal. Wilson was diagnosed with concussion and discharged that afternoon.

The day after the accident, Wilson felt pain in his neck, back, and head. He saw an orthopedic physician, who diagnosed him with whiplash injury. Several days later, Wilson saw a neurologist because he was having difficulty focusing, couldn't think clearly, had headaches, couldn't sleep, and felt anxious. His neurological exam was normal, as was a brain magnetic resonance imaging (MRI) scan. Wilson took several cognitive tests about a week after the accident and performed poorly on tests of processing speed and verbal memory. The neurologist determined that the sleep problems, headaches, and anxiety resulted from the concussion and recommended Tylenol (acetaminophen) as needed for the headaches. He educated Wilson about concussions and sleep hygiene, and suggested his patient take another week off from work. He did not prescribe any other medications.

Following the advice of his doctor, Wilson gradually resumed his usual activities, including work, doing the grocery shopping, and walking his dog, taking breaks as needed. He was relieved to find himself feeling back to normal in about six weeks. During this time, his symptoms (including his sleep, headaches, and anxiety) also gradually improved. According to his wife, he was "functioning as usual" about six weeks after the accident. He repeated the cognitive tests about two months after the accident and showed improvement on tests of information processing and verbal memory.

We examined brain structure and function in some detail in earlier chapters. We described different types of brain injury in chapter 3. In this chapter we explain how the brain can recover from injuries of various severity. Knowing how the brain recovers will help you understand the discussion in the next chapters of psychiatric symptoms following brain injury, because the behavioral interventions we suggest are based at least in part on brain recovery principles.

The brain is dynamic by nature, as it must be to make sense of a dynamic, changing world. There is inherent plasticity to the brain—that is, the brain can learn new ways of doing old things. This characteristic can help the brain recover from injury, as it enables us to train the brain using rehabilitation techniques.

The extent of recovery after brain injury depends on the severity of the injury. In cases of mild traumatic brain injury, for example, recovery within the first seven to ten days post-injury is typical, with full resolution of symptoms within a few months. A small percentage, about 10 to 15 percent of people, experience persistent symptoms. These persistent symptoms can be perpetuated by factors such as pain, stress and anxiety, poor sleep, or prolonged legal or insurance issues that frequently accompany TBIs. When perpetuating symptoms are addressed, persistent con-cussive symptoms are very likely to resolve.

In cases of moderate to severe brain injury, recovery may be slower and often depends on the nature of the injury, rehabilitation process, and support from family and friends. The pre-injury brain also determines a person's course of recovery. For example, an individual with trouble inhibiting behaviors pre-injury may be even more at risk post-injury for executive dysfunction (difficulty controlling impulses or emotions, and difficulty organizing and planning).

After a mild traumatic brain injury (also known as a concussion), people can experience physical symptoms (such as dizziness, headaches, sensitivity to light or sound), cognitive symptoms (usually problems with attention or memory), and mood symptoms (such as irritability, depression, or anxiety). People who have these symptoms may feel that they will never improve. The good news is that most people do in fact get better. Many people improve within days, and most within weeks to months. Wilson's recovery, in our opening story, is fairly typical of recovery from mild traumatic brain injury (TBI).

The rate of recovery varies from person to person, and certain types of symptoms improve more quickly than others. People will be more vulnerable to dizziness, for example, if the TBI affects the inner ear. Others may be more vulnerable to cognitive symptoms, such as inat-tention and slowed thinking. Some people who have many symptoms recover very quickly (within days), whereas others who have very few symptoms sometimes recover much more slowly.

Factors in Place before a Mild Brain Injury

A full recovery from a mild brain injury is almost always anticipated. But why is there variability in recovery? The exact nature of the injury plays a role, of course, but certain conditions affecting the person either before or after a mild brain injury can significantly affect their recovery.

Preexisting Mood or Emotional Disturbances

Preexisting mood or emotional disturbances can be a factor in recovering from a brain injury, so let's use anxiety as an example. If a person who suffers from anxiety suffers a mild brain injury, they may be at increased risk of becoming more anxious after the brain injury. Anxiety can increase because of the stress of suffering from the brain injury or because the injury affected circuits of the brain that control anxiety (for example, pain can create an increase in anxiety given how our brains are wired). The increase in anxiety can be obvious, making the person with the brain injury feel even more anxious, but it can also manifest in physical ways. The person with brain injury may be more sensitive to physical signals—slight dizziness or brief twinges of pain—that they might have ignored before their accident. They may have trouble concentrating and thus have problems with memory. These symptoms (such as memory problems) may initially be part of the brain injury, but anxiety can exacerbate or maintain them.

Mood problems that were present before a mild brain injury, like depression, can also affect the manifestation of symptoms after the injury. Depression can appear as slowness in thinking or problems with attention or memory, all of which could just as well be due to the brain injury. Depression, like anxiety, can worsen after mild brain injury. If depression (and anxiety) remains untreated after the injury, then recovery from symptoms ascribed to brain injury can be slow.

Depression may not only cause confusion as to what is due to the brain injury and what is due to other factors, but it may also directly influence recovery. For example, the person with depression may be less likely to follow up on rehabilitation or engage in behaviors, like exercise, that can facilitate recovery. Evidence from other neuropsychiatric conditions shows that depression may directly affect how the brain functions and recovers. Therefore, getting treatment for mood and anxiety symptoms after a brain injury can improve quality of life as well as improve recovery.

Alcohol and Substance Use

Another factor that can influence recovery from symptoms after brain injury is substance and alcohol use. Alcohol and other mind-altering substances (for example, cocaine, heroin, and marijuana) can directly impair the brain and thus impact recovery. These substances can also worsen mood and anxiety, thereby affecting the manifestation of symptoms. It is critical to avoid such substances to allow optimal recovery. In addition, abuse or misuse of pain pills (Percocet or Vicodin, for example) or tranquilizers (Valium, Xanax, Ativan) is not only dangerous, but can also interfere with recovery.

Overall Personality

Personality factors can also play a role in recovery after mild brain injury. Prominent anxiety traits may color how persons with brain injury perceive their improvement. In other words, even if an anxious person with brain injury is improving as expected, they may not be satisfied with their progress. Such thinking can prolong symptoms. Those with lifelong mood instability likewise can react catastrophically to a mild brain injury. Conversely, those who accept the mild brain injury as something that, while unfortunate, is not a catastrophe, typically recover more quickly.

Previous Brain Injuries

We now know that the number of previous brain injuries, at least traumatic brain injuries, can impact recovery. It may be harder to recover from the fourth TBI than the first. A series of even mild TBIs may lead to long-term impairment over the years in some individuals. Chronic traumatic encephalopathy (CTE) describes a condition that may develop in some individuals following accumulated damage from a series of mild TBIs. The few available studies suggest that CTE can manifest as behavioral or cognitive problems, with depression or dementia; and autopsies of patients who had CTE show characteristic physical damage to the brain. Research continues on CTE, but there is still a lot we do not know. What we do know is that multiple TBIs are not good for the brain, and having a history of multiple TBIs can adversely impact recovery.

Past Psychological Trauma

If a person with brain injury has had psychological trauma in the past or adverse childhood experiences, such as physical, emotional, or sexual abuse, an important aspect of recovery is how that person integrates the brain injury into their self-concept. Thinking about the brain injury less catastrophically may help with recovery. Being willing and able to participate in psychotherapy can help the person integrate the injury into their life story. Talking it out with family and friends can help with this, too. Practicing meditative and yoga techniques after brain injury may also be helpful in this process.

Factors in Place following a Brain Injury

Several critical factors after a brain injury can affect recovery. They include the following.

Supportive Social Network

Social support is an important factor in recovery. Although this fact may seem obvious, it is borne out by clinical experience and studies. Having a strong social network and family support can allow more time for rest, which is critical for optimal recovery. Emotional support from friends, family, and medical personnel may also directly affect the brain's ability to recover in ways that we do not yet understand.

Exercise

Lifestyle issues can affect recovery after a mild brain injury. Although it is important to rest and refrain from engaging in immediate athletic activity after a mild brain injury until cleared by a doctor, once cleared, exercise may help in various ways. In fact, increasing physical activity after a concussion is encouraged as long as it does not exacerbate symptoms. Exercise may improve mood and sleep, which in turn may alleviate symptoms. But it is important to develop a recovery plan based on recommendations by health care professionals.

Emotional State

Mood and anxiety symptoms that develop after mild brain injury can clearly impact recovery. In particular, post-traumatic stress disorder (PTSD) may develop after mild brain injury. The core symptoms of PTSD are reexperiencing the trauma (in nightmares or flashbacks), being on edge (being easily startled or irritable), and avoiding thinking about the trauma. PTSD may complicate recovery from symptoms after a brain injury, especially if the PTSD symptoms are not addressed directly. The symptoms can be hard to distinguish from mild TBI symptoms because some symptoms overlap, but clinicians with expertise in this area can manage the condition appropriately.

Legal Issues

Because a number of TBIs result from accidents where fault is often an issue, litigation and compensation can be factors impacting recovery, especially after a mild TBI. There will always be those who abuse the system and try to get compensation after TBI by exaggerating symptoms. Then there are others who truly have symptoms after a mild TBI. Sometimes symptoms may not be the direct result of TBI but may be associated with or exacerbated by the frustration and stress of dealing with the legal system, the police, or insurance companies. The impact of legal issues is commonly unintentional but can be significant. If your family member or you are dismissed by medical professionals or told they/you are "malingering" in order to benefit financially, you should consider obtaining a consultation with brain injury professionals.

A summary of the factors we have discussed relating to mild brain injuries appears in table 4.1.

TABLE 4.1. FACTORS THAT NEGATIVELY AND POSITIVELY IMPACT RECOVERY

Factors negatively influencing recovery	Factors positively influencing recovery
Preexisting mood or emotional problems	Supportive social network
Previous brain injuries	Exercise
Past psychological trauma	Emotional wellness
Personality traits such as inflexibility, impatience, impulsivity, rigidity, pessimism	Abstinence from alcohol and substance use
Stress from ongoing legal issues	Healthy diet and practicing relaxation exercises, for example, yoga or meditation

Recovery after Moderate to Severe Brain Injury

Recovery after a moderate to severe brain injury depends on a number of factors. Both the medical treatment received soon after the injury and the amount of brain tissue damage incurred affect the quality and success of recovery from severe brain injury. In most cases, immediate and appropriate medical or surgical treatment for conditions such as brain swelling or bleeding in the brain will increase the likelihood of a successful recovery. Similarly, the less damage to brain tissue, the greater the chance for recovery over time.

Rehabilitation plays a particularly large role in the immediate treatment of moderate to severe brain injury. Substantial physical, occupational, or cognitive rehabilitation is often necessary and beneficial. The quality of this rehabilitation, and the person's ability and willingness to undergo the rehabilitation, can affect recovery.

Of course, the severity of the brain injury is an important influence on recovery. The outlook is poor for those who are in a vegetative state after brain injury, meaning that they have lost meaningful cognitive function and awareness but continue breathing on their own.

Even among those with severe brain injury who are not in a vegetative state, long-term cognitive problems can impact recovery. There is some evidence that moderate to severe brain injury, at least traumatic brain injury, increases one's risk for developing Alzheimer's disease and Parkinson's disease, although not all studies support this theory.

As with mild brain injury, emerging mood, anxiety, and personality issues can affect optimal recovery after severe brain injury. Family and friends of persons who have experienced a severe brain injury may have to accept that the person with injury may never get back to the way they were prior to the injury. Accepting this "new baseline" can help the person integrate the consequences of their brain injury into their sense of self. However, it can be extremely challenging to develop a new sense of self when mourning one's pre-injury sense of self. If the person recovers only partially, the challenge is to help them achieve the best quality of life possible given their new circumstances. Psychotherapy and lifestyle practices like meditation can be effective tools in adjusting to "the new normal."

In this chapter, we covered a number of factors that affect recovery after brain injury. While it is obvious that persons with mild brain injury are more likely to recover fully, and faster, than those with moderate to severe brain injury, support from family and friends is important no matter what the severity of the injury. Persons with brain injury should be encouraged to seek and obtain the appropriate medical care, rehabilitation, brain injury support groups, and psychotherapy that makes sense for their post-injury needs. As we discussed earlier, mood issues such as anxiety and depression can make brain injury symptoms worse, and people should be encouraged to seek help for those common conditions. Family, friends, and caretakers of persons with brain injury have a critical role in helping them make sense of the trauma, both physical and psychological, accept what has happened, and consequently recover.

Take-Home Points

Full recovery is expected after a single mild brain injury.

Factors that interfere with recovery after mild brain injury include prior history of brain injury or injuries, alcohol and substance use before and after injury, mood and emotional problems before and after injury, ongoing insurance or litigation issues, and lack of social support.

Factors that interfere with recovery after moderate-to-severe brain injury include all of the above and the amount of brain tissue damage.

Part II

Neural Plasticity

In this part, we apply what we covered about the brain in part I. We focus on neural plasticity, the brain's ability to modify itself, discussing it in detail in chapters 5 and 6. It is useful to understand how the brain can change itself, and in doing so, help recovery after brain injury. We discuss a number of different methods that use the power of neural plasticity, including behavioral therapy (chapter 7), stress management techniques like meditation (chapter 8), cognitive training (chapter 9), and nutrition (chapter 10). We introduce these modalities now so that later in the book we can discuss their use in specific neuropsychiatric problems that develop after brain injury.

Chapter 5

The Idea
of Plasticity

When you hear the word *plastic*, it may give you an image of a container or a bag. But plastic also connotes flexibility and malleability. In the context of the brain, neural plasticity indicates the brain's ability to adjust, flex, reorganize itself, and form new connections and pathways in response to learning and experience.

If you think about it for a moment, your brain is always adjusting. It is always flexing to accommodate changes in the environment. For example, your eyes are moving all the time (these quick movements are called saccades). However, you don't see your environment moving with your eyes. Why is that? It's because your brain is adjusting for your eye movements and keeping your perception of the environment still.

Your brain is also always learning. Even if you are not engaged in formal learning in a school or class environment, your brain is always adjusting future expectations based on past experiences. For example, if you had a bad experience with being bitten by a dog in the past, chances are that you will learn to stay away from dogs. One of the major roles of the brain is to maximize chances of our survival, so learning what to avoid and what not to avoid is a critical aspect of what the brain does. Conversely, on a more positive note, our brain may learn that certain experiences, such as eating certain foods, or working hard at school and at work, give great pleasure and rewards, and the brain learns to seek out these experiences more.

Not so long ago, as recently as 40 years ago, scientists thought that the adult brain was not plastic; in other words, once you reached the age of 18, your brain was thought to be fully mature and only had a limited ability to adapt. At that time, the thinking was that children experience rapid brain growth and development, with dizzying amounts of neuronal production and synaptic growth, but adult brains were thought to be much less flexible or plastic. In other words, what you see by young adulthood is what you get. However, scientists have discovered since then that while it is true that children's brains have great plasticity, adults too can have significant brain plasticity and malleability.

While adults do not have the vast neuronal growth experienced by children, they too can experience growth and change in their brains, as adult brains can make new connections and pathways. In fact, learning (even in adulthood), is in essence making new connections and strengthening and changing certain synapses.

Brain injury leads to damage to brain circuits, but neuroplasticity is in a sense the reverse of damage to the brain: it is growth in the brain. In the next chapter we will discover more about neuroplasticity and how it can be leveraged to help heal the brain after injury.

TAKE-HOME POINTS

The brain is a dynamic organ with an inherent capacity to reorganize itself and form new connections.

Learning is a form of neuroplasticity.

Neuroplasticity can be potentially utilized to counter brain injury.

Chapter 6

Recovery from Brain Injury

As we discussed in chapter 5, neuroplasticity is the brain's ability to adjust, flex, reorganize itself, and form new connections and pathways in response to learning and repetition. As we now know, the brain is an extremely complex and dynamic organ. What may not be clear yet is that the brain creates our perceptions, and that ability is important in recovering from brain injury. That point is worth repeating: the brain actually creates our perceptions, our reality. How can this be? To understand, we have to step back and briefly discuss how we perceive and act on the world.

We know from our current understanding of physics that most of the reality we perceive in space is generated by the electromagnetic field, which is present everywhere, inside and outside our bodies. It is a quantum field (a field composed of quanta, or units of energy) that is changing constantly. The electromagnetic field contributes to our perception of light through our eyes, heat (infrared) through touch in various parts of our body, and sound through our ears in the form of radio waves that are converted to air pressure changes, which is what we perceive as sound. In short, reality as we perceive it is due mainly to this field.

What we perceive in the brain are excitations of this field—or to be more accurate, what we perceive is the model of this field created by the brain. For example, what we perceive and label as light is actually rapid vibrations of the electromagnetic field. When you open your eyes and see someone, what you are really seeing are rapid vibrations of the electromagnetic field entering your eye. Higher frequencies in the visible spectrum are perceived as indigo and blue, while lower frequencies are perceived as yellow and red. Colors are what our brain creates from the data it gets from a quantum field.

A brain injury (such as a stroke) can cause unilateral (one-sided) damage that can leave a gap in perception or awareness. In this condition, we may not be aware of one part of our own body or a sector of space; such a condition is called unilateral spatial neglect. Losing awareness of a section of space can be a very difficult problem after stroke, as the person cannot participate in rehabilitation properly when they are not even aware of their weak limb. But how can someone lose awareness that their own body part exists? This loss occurs because the brain's representation of the sector of space where the limb is becomes damaged. In this way, the body is a projection of the brain—the brain creates the representation of the body and projects it "out there" in space.

Another way to think about all of this is that reality as we perceive it is literally in our brains. We cannot get outside our own brains. When people dismiss or downplay our concerns and say that "it must be in your head," that is more accurate (in a different way) than they probably know. The brain translates sensory input into electrical patterns and uses those patterns to plan and move and think. The patterns are the currency of the brain, and everything we perceive and act on is also via the brain—there are no colors or shapes or sounds in the brain, only electrical patterns.

Understanding that the brain creates our reality is important to understand brain injury, as our reality can change when our brains are injured. Our perceptions, our movements, our moods, our attention, our memory, our thinking, and our very behavior can all be changed when there is damage to the brain.

On the other hand, understanding that our brain is plastic, malleable, and changeable can provide hope for recovery after brain injury.

Our brains are always changing, and change can improve things after a brain injury. Injured areas of the brain can be bypassed by other neural circuits. As we have already discussed, the brain includes circuits that are devoted to certain tasks, and there definitely are circuits that are specialized. However, after a brain injury, other circuits can be recruited to compensate for injured circuits. This process is not easy or immediate, but it is possible. As the writer Will Durant wrote, paraphrasing Aristotle, we are what we repeatedly do. Practicing tasks and repeating activities can help with rewiring the brain. Similarly, it is possible that enriching our lives with novelty, creativity, and challenges can promote neuroplasticity.

It is important to note that recovery involves significant effort on the part of the person who has had brain injury. Harnessing neuroplasticity to recover from brain injury can involve medications, talk therapy, stress management, and self-care techniques like meditation and yoga, brain training via games, proper sleep, physical exercise—and likely in the near future, brain stimulation techniques such as using magnets to directly activate parts of the brain. Simple healthy activities that are nourishing for the brain and have the potential to rewire it are listed in table 6.1.

TABLE 6.1. STRATEGIES TO ENHANCE NEUROPLASTICITY
Exercising regularly
Eating a healthy diet of fruits, vegetables, whole grains, proteins; hydrating adequately
Quitting tobacco and street drugs; reducing or eliminating alcohol
Engaging in hobbies
Staying active by learning new tasks as long as they are pleasurable
Practicing relaxation and self-care (such as yoga and meditation)
Practicing sleep hygiene (see chapter 20)

All these techniques may work by stimulating undamaged neurons, leading to increased connections between them, in effect rewiring circuits so that they can compensate for areas that are damaged. There is a saying in neuroscience that "neurons that fire together wire together." When two neurons are repetitively fired together, changes occur in the synapse between the two neurons to allow them to fire with less stimulation in the future. Imagine a hiking path that becomes well worn, so that hikers can eventually travel the path with more ease as more travelers walk upon it. Practice and repetition are critical until the new circuits are stabilized, because it is also true that neuroplasticity can go in the opposite direction too—as the saying goes, use it or lose it.

Not all plasticity is favorable. We may, for example, remember negative thoughts and experiences too well and overlearn the lessons they teach us. Experiencing pain chronically for many years is a good example of lessons overlearned. In people who experience chronic pain, their brain has become very sensitive to events or activities perceived by them as uncomfortable or distressing. In such cases, everyday life activities such as dressing, showering, or doing simple house chores can cause or worsen baseline pain. As a result, someone living with chronic pain learns to avoid these activities, which can be unhealthy and unproductive and even cause secondary pain due to inactivity. Another example of the downside of brain plasticity is phantom limb syndrome. In this condition, people who have lost a limb may still feel the limb (it is a "phantom limb") because the brain's representation of the limb is still there even though the limb itself is gone. Worse still, in some cases, the representation of the missing limb flexes and merges with the representation of a body part that is intact; for example, touching the face may lead to pain in the missing limb.

As another example, people with social anxiety disorder may be uncomfortable physically in social situations, and so they avoid those situations. Unfortunately, that avoidance can lead to perpetuating the problem. However, with the right kind of therapy, they will be able to learn other strategies to improve their social skills. With traumatic events, people can develop post-traumatic stress disorder (PTSD), which can occur in conjunction with brain injury, as the event that caused the brain injury can be traumatizing at a psychological level. This disorder can lead to very vivid memories of the trauma, with physical signs related to the stress response every time the memories come up. These memories and physical responses can in turn lead to anxiety and avoidance of situations or places that call up the memories. Just as in social anxiety disorder, this avoidance can lead to perpetuation of the problem, which can be treated with a combination of medications and therapy. Therapy can help people unlearn their negative thinking and learn new behaviors to cope with anxiety-producing situations.

Despite the potential downsides, brain plasticity does demonstrate that the brain can change, and can change quite dramatically. Unfortunately, the negative effects of a brain injury can be fast and automatic, and to get the benefits of brain plasticity, repeated effort and time is usually needed to undo any negative learning. Nonetheless, understanding plasticity can help the person with brain injury help themselves recover. Harnessing the brain's inherent plasticity can be very helpful in surviving and even at some point thriving. Among the numerous techniques that can help support the positive benefits of brain plasticity are cognitive behavioral therapy (a kind of psychotherapy focused on identifying and changing negative thinking patterns and behavior), cognitive rehabilitation (such as memory or attention adaptation training), brain stimulation techniques (such as transcranial magnetic stimulation), medications, meditation, or even engaging in new pleasurable hobbies or exercises. Another good example is visual rehabilitation in persons with visual field defects. Clinicians experienced in this field train people with this defect on eye scanning movements to compensate for visual loss or improve vision using techniques to activate residual, or remaining, visual functions. All these rehabilitation strategies enhance and capitalize on neuroplasticity.

Take-Home Points

The brain is malleable and has the potential to reorganize itself and strengthen new pathways.

Repeated practice of tasks/activities can help in learning the task and retraining the brain.

Enriched and stimulating environments can help with neuroplasticity.

Chapter 7

Behavioral Therapy

M any people have heard of, participated in, or know someone who has participated in, talk therapy. Talk therapy (also known as psychotherapy) includes behavioral or cognitive techniques. The general theme is to engage with someone at a conversational level to facilitate change. Talk therapy targets both a person's thoughts (cognitions) and behaviors, ultimately potentially causing long-term changes in the brain using neuroplasticity.

There are several different types of psychotherapies, which include a number of evidence-based approaches, such as cognitive behavioral therapy and motivational interviewing. Many evidence-based psychotherapies are relatively structured, though they have the flexibility to be adapted to rehabilitation populations, such as individuals who have cognitive challenges due to a brain injury. It may not always be clear how therapy can help an individual when it seems memory or attention problems would prevent them from benefiting. For instance, how would a person with insomnia after brain injury benefit from therapy when the person is having significant memory problems? However, adapting therapies to address targeted issues is commonly done within the rehabilitation setting. Even for more severe brain injuries, some form of psychotherapeutic intervention (at times calling upon the family) can be of benefit. In those cases, behaviorally focused interventions may be useful.

Even individuals with significant cognitive challenges due to a severe brain injury can engage in and benefit from a therapeutic alliance that fosters honesty and trust. It is not uncommon for those whose injury imposed impaired awareness to make positive changes in their lives and behaviors, not necessarily because of a powerful insight developed in therapy, but because they trust the therapist and believe that person is in their corner.

Therapists use different approaches to improve relationships with their patients to help them change their behavior and adopt healthy living strategies. Motivational interviewing (MI) is one such evidence-based approach that includes evaluation and counseling via multiple sessions to motivate the person to adopt helpful and healthy coping and compensatory strategies that are consistent with their values.

As a concrete example, consider an individual living with a brain injury who insists that he is going to leave his cane behind on a trip to a local park. His lack of insight regarding his poor balance and the risk of another brain injury makes it difficult for him to make a decision in his best interest. A psychologist trained in working with individuals who have incurred brain injury can work with him using MI techniques to elicit positive behavioral change without confrontation. In this case, as the person continues to argue with the psychologist against using the cane, the psychologist notes to the patient the importance of not getting injured and the fact that being without a cane can lead to injury. The patient, however, says that he does not care if he gets injured. With this information, the psychologist changes course and helps the patient to identify what he does value. In this case, he values seeing his grandchildren play soccer. With that as the goal, the psychologist and patient work collaboratively—not confrontationally—on moving him toward using a cane so that his behavior is in line with his values. That is, the psychologist points out that, given the patient's values, he would be able to get to his grandchildren's soccer game more easily if he uses his cane.

For milder brain injuries, talk therapy can be quite helpful, both to help target issues and to help the person with the injury best manage their new situation. Cognitive behavioral therapy (CBT) is well established as an effective treatment for addressing cognitive distortions (unrealistic negative thoughts about the present situation and the future) in the general population as well as among individuals who have incurred a brain injury. The concept of CBT is that our thoughts, emotions, and behaviors are interconnected, and the technique is aimed at addressing unhelpful thoughts and behaviors. By targeting one's thoughts (such as loss of sense of self) and behaviors (such as decreased involvement in fun activities), shifts in emotions such as anxiousness, hopelessness, or depression can occur. An important concept in CBT is that our thoughts may not all be helpful. One technique to target unhelpful thoughts is to learn how to "think like a scientist." That is, in observing our thoughts, what is the evidence for the thought, and what is the evidence against the thought?

In major depression, for example, there can be a cognitive bias where negative, unhelpful thoughts are more prominent. In CBT, one learns to examine these automatic negative thoughts and judge their validity. It is not that we want all our thoughts to be positive (although that would be great). It is that we want to shift unhelpful thoughts to more realistic or helpful ones. For example, the thought that "I am broken and am never going to be the same" shifts to "I had an injury that has changed my life in many ways, some for the better and some not."

The behavioral part of CBT can involve facilitating certain behaviors to help frame thoughts in a more realistic manner. For example, if someone is having symptoms of a panic attack—their heart is racing and they think they may be having a heart attack—a behaviorally focused technique would be to have the person run up and down stairs (thereby increasing heart rate) and demonstrating that they are not causing a heart attack (after making sure, of course, that they do not in fact have heart problems).

Other types of behavioral therapies that have been shown to have some effectiveness in persons with brain injury include behavioral activation therapy and acceptance and commitment therapy. Behavioral activation focuses on replacing negative unhealthy behaviors with new rewarding behaviors with the goal of maintaining and reinforcing healthy behaviors. Acceptance and commitment therapy uses strategies from mindfulness of accepting suffering/pain/negative feelings, choosing behaviors as defined by the person's values, and making a commitment to change.

Behavioral approaches can also be more subtle. Attention to behaviors tends to magnify those behaviors. Attending to and praising positive behaviors tend to increase those behaviors, while attending to and criticizing negative behaviors may actually make them worse. For a caregiver to a person with a more severe brain injury, a behavioral approach may work best. They could create a list of positive behaviors and negative behaviors that their brain-injured loved one is engaging in. They could then consciously focus on attending to the positive behaviors. Such a treatment plan includes concrete reinforcement of positive behaviors, whereby the person with brain injury gets a reward of some sort with more of these positive behaviors. With inappropriate behaviors, the caregiver could minimize their reaction to the behaviors (after assuring their own safety). Over time, the inappropriate behaviors will tend to decrease or extinguish without the oxygen of attention.

There are other types of psychotherapies that can be helpful based on particular situations. For example, for a person with a brain injury who is facing difficulty with family relationships, a form of interpersonal therapy may be helpful, focusing on strategies to increase interpersonal efficacy, with better understanding of the needs of everyone and better communication about those needs.

Ultimately, psychotherapy involves learning. Working with a clinician over time, if effective, leads to learning how to think or act differently in line with one's core values and goals. Learning involves brain plasticity. In fact, one of the most prominent types of neural plasticity, long-term potentiation (LTP), is critical in learning. LTP is based on the notion that if a neuron gets a pattern of input to it repeatedly over time, the neuron sensitizes to that input, and in the future it is more likely to fire. Ultimately this is what learning is—we associate something with something else (the letter *n* with its particular sound, for example). At a neuronal level, over time, the association becomes more and more automatic. At a behavioral level, the association also becomes more and more automatic. After learning the sound that *n* makes, we do not have to think about it: it is now automatic. We have learned it.

It is because our brain is changeable and malleable that therapy can help after brain injury. Even though it may seem that talking may not have brain effects, that is not the case. Talking ultimately can lead to learning, and learning is a brain process. Luckily, even after a brain injury, we can take advantage of this process.

TAKE-HOME POINTS

Psychotherapy, including CBT, involves learning and has the potential to help increase neuroplasticity.

Talk with your health care professional about the most appropriate type of therapy for you given your particular problems.

Most rehabilitation programs are staffed with rehabilitation neuro-psychologists and social workers who can help establish a therapy plan.

Chapter 8

Stress Management

A term we use all the time is *stress*. Everyone knows intuitively what it is, but it can be surprisingly difficult to define. That could be because what is stressful for one person may not be stressful for someone else. For example, bungee jumping may be incredibly stressful for some, while it can be exhilarating for others. What is stressful is very individualized. Nevertheless, one definition could be that stress occurs when the demands of a task overwhelm our cognitive resources.

With brain injury, cognitive resources may be more limited, and what was not stressful before can become stressful now. Before brain injury, getting ready in the morning, for instance, may have been routine and not particularly stressful. But after a brain injury, the same task may be very stressful. Stress management, then, while important for everyone, may be particularly important for persons with brain injury and those that care for them.

One stress management tool, meditation, can be helpful for anyone, but especially for those living with brain injury, as well as caregivers. There is increasing evidence that meditation may be correlated with cognitive capacities such as attention, as well as increased neuroplasticity.

There are various ways to conceptualize and engage in meditation. Meditation is rooted in practices that evolved thousands of years ago in India. In this chapter, we focus on two types that have some of the greatest evidence of success in managing stress. Mindfulness meditation is one such type of meditation. Mindfulness has been researched within the context of physical and mental health over the years and has gained growing support as to its efficacy.

Mindfulness is based on the premise that our brains are often thinking about the past or worrying about the future but are not so much in the present moment. That is, attention is not focused on the here and now. The goal of mindfulness meditation is to train the brain to be more in the present, based on the idea that present-centered awareness leads to improved quality of life.

One way to train the brain in mindfulness is to listen to and follow guided meditations. Guided meditations are available online and often involve focusing on one part of the body or sequentially focusing on different parts of the body. For example, you might be encouraged to sit or lie quietly and be guided to focus first on your feet, perhaps tensing and then relaxing, working your way up through the body to the head, neck, and face. Another method is to simply focus on the breathing. Yet another method is to have a mantra (a word or phrase) that you focus the mind on. When you are aware that your mind has wandered off, you gently bring it back to what you were doing (either following a guided meditation or your mantra or being aware of your breathing). Your mind will likely wander off again—and again, you bring your awareness back to what you were doing. The key is to do this repeatedly without judgment, and without getting mad at yourself for getting off track, as agitation just makes it harder to get back to the meditation or mantra you were doing.

Another form of mindfulness is open awareness (often known as vipassana), where you are allowing yourself to have thoughts like normal, but you are not judging them or delving into them. It is like watching clouds go by in the sky—you just watch the clouds; you don't dive into them. This open awareness can be done as part of a daily practice but can also be done while engaging in daily life (like taking a walk, for example).

Mindfulness meditation is quite simple conceptually, though the key is to follow through and practice it gently and on a regular basis. It is best to do it daily, perhaps 10 to 15 (or more) minutes a day. Though the time while you are practicing may be beneficial by itself, there can be long-term benefit as well. In the long term, mindfulness meditation may increase your stress buffering, your ability to withstand stressors and maintain your equilibrium.

Transcendental meditation (TM) is another technique that uses a mantra, but it does not involve concentrating on the mantra. This technique has a significant evidence base, showing unique brain changes, as well as significant benefit for depression, anxiety, and general physical health (decreased blood pressure, decreased blood sugar, and even decreased risk for strokes and heart attacks). Practiced for 20 minutes twice a day, TM also seems to help with stress buffering, like mindfulness. The American Heart Association, for example, recommends TM for high blood pressure patients (and has suggested meditation in general as a reasonable adjunct for cardiac patients). The downside to TM is that it is not as easily accessible as mindfulness, since there is a financial cost associated with mastering it, because the TM organization charges for teaching the technique.

Besides meditation, other techniques that involve more physical activity might be beneficial for those living with brain injury and their caregivers, particularly yoga. Yoga has become immensely popular over time in the United States, and many cities now have yoga studios. Just as there are various forms of meditation, there are various forms of yoga, all originating from ancient India. We focus on two types of yoga, both with significant studies to support their use.

Hatha yoga is what most people think about when they hear the word *yoga*. Hatha yoga involves doing and maintaining specific postures, something that can be quite challenging physically, and so may not be feasible for every person living with a brain injury. It is important to practice yoga under guidance and with care. If necessary, a teacher can suggest modified postures and guide you through them. Yoga often involves mindfulness, as well, since keeping your mind on your breathing and on the particular posture you are doing is encouraged. Over the past few years, yoga teachers and studios have begun to offer classes specifically for individuals who have experienced a brain injury and are able to modify poses for those living with significant physical challenges and conditions related to brain injury.

Another kind of yoga is rhythmic breathing yoga, including Sudarshan Kriya Yoga (SKY). SKY involves breathing at different rhythms for set periods of time, from slow, to medium, to fast. Mindful attending is encouraged while engaging in the breathing rhythms. SKY has been studied and shown to reduce depression, anxiety, and traumatic stress symptoms in various conditions.

We have discussed meditation and yoga so far mostly in the context of stress relief. And, indeed, a brain injury can be a very stressful and even traumatic experience (with some patients developing post-traumatic stress disorder, or PTSD). Adapting to a new normal, potentially with new restrictions on what is doable, can be very stressful. Those living with brain injury, as well as their caretakers and supporters, can have stress related to the behavioral, mood, or cognitive changes in their lives. For all these reasons, having meditation and yoga techniques in your self-care toolkit can be very beneficial.

Beyond these benefits, there is also the possibility that these techniques can help cause beneficial brain changes and improve certain types of cognitive faculties such as attention/concentration and working memory (a type of immediate memory) due to improved neural plasticity. Brain imaging studies in long-time meditators provide evidence that physical brain growth occurs (with increased connections between brain areas). There is also evidence of changes in blood flow patterns or electrical connectivity, generally causing increased efficiency of brain processing. TM in particular has a large body of evidence suggesting increased coherence in alpha brain waves in the frontal lobes, which could be beneficial for cognitive functioning and mood regulation.

While there have not been many studies of meditation (or yoga) for brain injury, we do have evidence from the general population and from patients suffering from neuropsychiatric disorders (including major depression, generalized anxiety disorder, mild cognitive impairment, PTSD, and obsessive-compulsive disorder) that there may be a benefit from these techniques. Given that they are unlikely to cause any harm, and given their potential for benefit, learning these techniques may be a useful addition to your brain injury recovery toolkit.

<hr>

Take-Home Points

Meditation is for all but can be especially helpful for persons with brain injury and their caregivers.

There are many types of meditation; mindfulness-based meditation and TM have the potential to be effective for persons with brain injury but need to be studied further.

Meditation has many benefits. It can help to improve physical health, emotional health, and cognitive faculties.

<hr>

Exercise

Although it is best to learn meditation from a professional, you can start by doing one or more of these exercises. Remember, starting your day mindfully will help you to have a better day.

• *The goal of mindfulness is to try to be in the present moment without judging yourself or the moment and without trying to change the experience. Commonly, this is done by setting an intention to do something or pay attention to something specific, like focusing on your breathing, or the sounds you hear, the thoughts going through your mind, the sensation on your skin, or the taste of what you are eating. Then, just notice that experience. Pay attention to the details. If you notice that your mind wanders off, you are doing it right—noticing that your mind wandered is being mindful. The exercise then is to observe that your mind trailed off, and then kindly, nonjudgmentally, guide yourself back to what you had set your intention to do. The exercise itself* is the bringing back of your attention. It is not refusing to allow your mind to go. Over time, you will notice that your ability to pay attention and focus improves.

• Find a comfortable, quiet place and practice a simple breathing exercise. Close your eyes and breathe in slowly through your nose to a count of 5, and breathe out through your mouth to a count of 7. Repeat this exercise a few times. If you are distracted by noises or anything else around you, make a mental note of the distraction, allow it to pass, and come back to your breathing. Notice any urges that arise to silence the distraction and allow those urges to pass too.

• If you like taking walks, find a quiet place to walk. As you walk, pay attention to your balance, your steps, and your movements. Experience other sensations around you as they come and go, but continue to focus on your walk.

• If you are having a stressful, busy day, take about a 10- to 15-minute break at the end of every hour and do something fun such as coloring, flipping through a magazine, walking around the room, listening to music, or even simply closing your eyes and just focusing on your body sensations, such as pain, temperature, touch, itch, or any other sensation.

• Start your day by having a simple goal or intention for the day. For example, tell yourself, "I will try to act peacefully, calmly, and not get angry." As you go through the day, keep a check of how often you were able to stay calm rather than losing your temper. It does not matter what the counts are. Try not to judge or berate yourself. But with time, as you pay attention to the goal you set, you will come closer to attaining it.

• Chant a mantra. Find a quiet, comfortable place to sit. Choose your favorite word or syllable (or a mantra given to you by a med-

itation teacher). Close your eyes and repeat the word for about five minutes. You can do so silently or aloud. As you do, be aware of the vibrations of your lips, and mouth, and other bodily sensations. If your mind wanders as you chant, take a short pause and then kindly guide your mind back to your chant.

Chapter 9

Cognitive Rehabilitation

Fifty-eight-year-old Fred was doing well as a computer programmer until he had a sudden stroke that affected the left side of his brain and caused weakness on his right side, including his upper and lower limbs, and difficulties with speech, predominantly with expressing himself. He was admitted to the stroke unit of a large hospital. About 72 hours later, he was transferred to the acute rehabilitation facility in the same hospital. Here, he underwent a thorough evaluation by a multidisciplinary team, including a physiatrist, neuropsychologist, occupational therapist, speech-language pathologist, and physical therapist. Each one of these clinicians focused on different aspects of his problems—the physiatrist on his medical issues, the neuropsychologist on his cognition, the physical therapist on his gait and balance, the occupational therapist on his ability to do everyday tasks, and the speech-language pathologist on his speech and language. The evaluation was followed by regular treatment by the various clinicians in a coordinated way with weekly multidisciplinary meetings. Fred was compliant with treatment and gradually made progress. By the end of six weeks, he was able to walk steadily using a walker, was able to take care of his personal activities such as feeding, showering, and dressing, and was able to communicate (though he still had word-finding problems). He was discharged from the inpatient rehabilitation facility at the end of six weeks. However, he continued to have mood and cognitive issues, such as easy anger and irritability, quickly reacting to situations without thinking through them. He also had difficulties working on complex tasks, such as tasks that required more than two steps and tasks that required organizing, planning, and prioritizing. These difficulties greatly interfered with his ability to maintain his job and interact with his family and friends, causing significant stress in the family. He continued outpatient rehabilitation with the same multidisciplinary team for another few months. He continued to make gradual progress, and by the end of one year, he was able to better interact with family and friends. Fred also rejoined work, at first part-time, and a few months later, full-time. He no longer required speech-language, physical, or occupational therapies, but continued to have biweekly sessions with the rehabilitation neuropsychologist for management of residual behavioral and cognitive issues such as impulsivity and difficulty organizing and executing tasks.

As we have discussed in previous chapters, neural plasticity is critical for recovering from a brain injury, and learning is a form of plasticity. Whenever we learn something, we cause physical changes in our brain: our neural connections change when we learn. Changing neural connections translates into neurons firing in a different pattern, a physical alteration of the brain's function.

Cognitive rehabilitation is one way to harness the power of learning. The goal of cognitive rehabilitation is to set goals, learn compensation techniques, master those compensatory techniques, and then generalize them (apply them to everyday life). Cognitive rehabilitation can be thought of as a means of facilitating remediation (recovery) and developing compensation (managing the dysfunction). It's like a kind of exercise to capitalize on plasticity. Just like we need to repeatedly do (practice) physical exercises to cause changes in our body, we can repeatedly do (practice) cognitive exercises and ways of compensating to cause changes in our brain.

If a brain injury has caused cognitive problems such as poor attention, impulse control, or memory, we can practice those skills to improve them, or more often, to compensate for them. Using a framework implemented by a multidisciplinary team is important and can include neuropsychiatrists, rehabilitation neuropsychologists, speech-language pathologists, physical therapists, and occupational therapists. The key is to establish a multipronged plan of care based on the individual's challenges and strengths. A comprehensive evaluation is absolutely necessary prior to treatment of cognitive problems to determine and treat all potential contributory factors including general medical issues (such as seizures) and psychiatric issues (such as clinical depression).

An example of how cognitive rehabilitation works can be seen in the case from the beginning of the chapter. The stroke to the left side of the brain caused Fred multiple deficits: right-sided physical weakness, speech and language difficulties, and problems with executive function. The team of clinicians, each of whom had expertise in a specific domain, worked with Fred to improve his deficits.

Cognitive rehabilitation strategies that the neuropsychologist used successfully with Fred included metacognitive training and problem-solving training. Metacognitive training (which is basically thinking about thinking) can be helpful in managing impulsive responding. The goal is to teach someone to stop their impulsive response, predict how they will do on a task, complete the task, review how they did, and then report how they did. Then, with feedback, improved monitoring of behavior can occur. Problem-solving training includes working with the therapist to define the problem, determine other factors related to the problem, generate various possible solutions to the problem, identify pros and cons associated with the various solutions, choose and follow a solution that has the greatest potential to get the best result, and finally evaluate the results.

Cognitive rehabilitation has evidence-based guidelines that can help drive treatment. For example, attentional problems can be addressed with attention process training, and executive functioning problems may be managed with metacognitive training. The overarching goal of rehabilitation therapy is to help the person maximize recovery and adjust, adapt, and learn strategies to cope with any injury-imposed barriers so they can attain their goals for their own lives, at home, at work, and in the community.

More recently, computer-based games have been developed with the notion that they might help facilitate cognitive recovery. Although there have been some interesting findings in relation to the games, it may be too soon to know if they have clinical utility for brain injury, since it is not clear how they impact everyday functions. In some disorders, the benefits are more well established, such as ADHD (attention-deficit/hyperactivity disorder), with the US Food and Drug Administration (FDA) clearing a prescription computer-based game for ADHD in children.

We are still awaiting results from more research studies to inform us of the effectiveness, success, and challenges associated with digital therapeutic games. Until then, cognitive rehabilitation within a rehabilitation program is the gold standard of treatment—programs that are multidisciplinary and include a focus on cognitive and emotional functions. Cognitive rehabilitation techniques paired with psychotherapeutic interventions to elicit awareness are likely to facilitate the best outcome. Such interventions are the springboard for skills, with repetition allowing for enhanced neuroplasticity. With practice and guidance, maximal recovery can be achieved.

Take-Home Points

A comprehensive evaluation is an important aspect of treatment of cognitive challenges following brain injury to help determine if there are other contributory factors that are posing barriers to the individual as they work toward their goals and recovery.

A one-size-fits-all approach will not work. Treatment needs be tailored to the specific needs of the individual and in coordination with that person and their support system, such as family.

Cognitive rehabilitation involves the remediation of cognitive challenges (such as attention training early on in recovery) and compensation (such as using a planner to write down information) when memory is impaired. For the person with brain injury, it is important to continue to practice at home the exercises and strategies learned from the therapist. Working with professionals to maintain integration of skills is important and should be part of the rehabilitation program.

Exercise

Therapy should be individualized, but here are a few general things that anyone having cognitive challenges can consider doing:

- *Have fun while learning—buddy up with someone who is part of your support system and play games such as card and board games.*

- *Challenge yourself by playing mental games such as crossword puzzles, Sudoku, picture puzzles, word-search puzzles, and so forth.*

- *Try to do something different—for example, use your non-dominant hand (left hand if you are a right-handed person) to write or color. You can even try brushing your teeth with your non-dominant hand for an additional challenge!*

- *Keep a schedule with the use of a paper calendar or smartphone. Block the day into time slots and plan a structured routine. For example, eat meals at the same time each day and go for a walk at the same time.*

- *Pace your activities. Focus on one step at a time. Avoid multitasking.*

Chapter 10

Nutrition

In much of the world now, a diet with significant amounts of processed and sugary foods has become predominant. Unfortunately, such a diet is not very good for brain health. This is because our brain, like the rest of our body, needs proper sources of energy. In fact, our brain needs more energy proportionately than the rest of our body. The brain is about 5 percent of total body weight, but it takes up about 25 percent of the body's energy needs. It is all the more important that we focus on nutrition after a brain injury because energy needs are so important to the brain.

What is good for the heart is usually good for the brain. The reason is that good blood flow from the heart to the brain is critical for good brain functioning. Good blood flow and hence good blood vessel health is critical for getting energy to the brain.

Brain injury can lead to inflammation, which can cause damage to blood vessels. Inflammation is one of the ways that your immune system attempts to deal with injury. Unfortunately, with a brain injury, inflammation can make the injury worse. Our diet can also be pro-inflammatory. Processed foods with high sugar content and high-fat foods can cause more inflammation. Foods that have anti-inflammatory properties include fresh fruits, green leafy vegetables, fish such as salmon, and certain nuts and oils.

The Mediterranean diet encompasses a number of anti-inflammatory foods. It emphasizes fruits, vegetables, lean meats, nuts, and olive oil.

Several clinical studies suggest that such a diet may help with cardiac and brain health.

There are also variants of the Mediterranean diet, which focus on fruits and vegetables (such as the Nutritarian diet). Whether you choose to follow a specific diet plan or just change your diet to include more vegetables, fruits, whole grains, and lean meat, as recommended by the American Heart Association (see the exercise below), it is important that you stay consistent and keep up with healthy eating on a daily basis. You might even wish to consult with a nutritionist, who can help guide you in making healthy choices around food.

The focus of the diets we have discussed—fruits and vegetables—can also be understood from a physics point of view. Life is ultimately a process of fighting entropy (disorder or disorganization). We have to expend energy to keep our bodies from becoming more disordered. We do this by tapping into a source of low entropy and high energy, the sun, which provides us the organization for our bodies to fight decay. Plants convert the sun's energy via chlorophyll to energy (and low entropy) that we can consume.

A plant-based diet is thus a direct way to tap into the sun's energy and its organizing effects on our body. Eating plant-based foods is a good way to efficiently improve energy availability for the brain. Doing so is important especially after a brain injury, which can lead to increased energy demands for the brain. Highly processed foods provide much less of the sun's energy than fruits and vegetables, and thus, they do not have the same benefits for our brain and body in staving off entropy or disorganization.

Improved energy access for the brain can help it recover after an injury. Neural plasticity, as we have discussed, is critical for brain injury recovery—and plasticity involves significant energy expenditure, because the brain has to create new connections. Having a good source of efficient energy is thus critical to maximize chances and rates of recovery.

What we eat can also affect our microbiome, the repository of (mostly) bacteria in our gut, bacteria that actually outnumber human cells. Over recent years, it has become more apparent that the microbiome plays a critical role in our health. It can affect our kidney functioning, blood sugar levels, and our blood pressure. Even more surprisingly, the microbiome may modulate our immune system and our inflammatory response, which can affect our brain. Indeed, there are studies that show the microbiome might modulate mood and anxiety levels.

What we eat is critical to what bacteria thrive in our microbiome. As it turns out, fruits and vegetables are good sources for healthy bacteria in our microbiome. High-fiber foods (such as green leafy vegetables) provide nutrients for these healthy bacteria, which then increase in quantity. The healthy bacteria can then predominate over less healthy bacteria, affecting our microbiome balance in a good way. Processed, high-sugar, and high-fat foods modulate the balance in our microbiome in the opposite direction, thus potentially causing more problems for our body, including our brain.

Nutrition is important for our health in general, but particularly for brain health. With the proper diet, people with brain injuries can help meet their brain's energy needs and also improve their overall health (particularly heart health). Good nutrition can also lead to weight loss for those who are overweight, or can help maintain appropriate weight if not overweight. It can also decrease inflammation—which can lead to improved mood and improved cognition (such as attention and memory). Of course, it is impractical to eat only healthful foods all the time, but trying to maximize the proportion of what we eat that has high nutrient value can be well worth the effort, especially after a brain injury.

Take-Home Points

Brain injury can lead to inflammation. The consumption of processed foods with high sugar and high fat content can also cause inflammation. Therefore, an anti-inflammatory diet is very important during recovery.

What is good for the heart is usually good for the brain.

Diets rich in fruits and vegetables have anti-inflammatory properties and are good for the brain.

Exercise

Follow the recommendations of the American Heart Association: eat at least eight servings of fruits and vegetables per day for a 2,000-calorie diet. The fruits and vegetables can be fresh, frozen, canned, or dried. However, avoid excess salt and sugar.

Check out these American Heart Association websites for more information on adding fruits and vegetables to your diet:

- *"Fruits and Vegetables Serving Sizes Infographic," https://www.heart.org/en/healthy-living/healthy-eating/add-color/fruits-and-vegetables-serving-sizes*

- *"All Colors, All the Time," https://www.heart.org/en/healthy-living/healthy-eating/add-color*

- *"How to Eat More Fruit and Vegetables," https://www.heart.org/en/healthy-living/healthy-eating/add-color/how-to-eat-more-fruits-and-vegetables*

Emotional Problems Caused *by the* Traumatized Brain

In part I, we discussed the structure and function of the brain. In part II, we applied that knowledge to discover how neuroplasticity may help in recovery from brain injury. In part III, we start to delve into specific neuropsychiatric consequences of brain injury, especially emotional symptoms after brain injury. We explore depression (chapter 11), mania (chapter 12), anxiety (chapter 13), and PTSD (post-traumatic stress disorder) (chapter 14), problems that can significantly impact quality of life and recovery from brain injury.

Depression

At 33, John was a successful carpenter working on a construction site when he fell from a ladder 40 feet to the ground. When he didn't regain consciousness after the fall, his coworkers called an ambulance, which sped him to the nearest hospital. Brain scans revealed that John was bleeding in the right and left frontal lobes and the left temporal lobe. He remained in a coma in the intensive care unit for two weeks. His doctors monitored his brain swelling and vital signs and decided against performing brain surgery because the bleeding was gradually resolving.

Three weeks after his fall, John was alert and gradually regaining his ability to care for himself. He could mostly feed himself, go to the bathroom, and get dressed with little help from the hospital staff. He was transferred to an inpatient rehabilitation unit, where he received speech and language therapy, physical therapy, and occupational therapy. After a month of rehabilitation, he was better able to get around on his own and independently take care of his personal hygiene and grooming. John was discharged from the hospital and continued to receive outpatient occupational, physical, and speech and language therapy for the next six months.

Soon after John came home, his family and friends noticed that he was just not the same person he had been before the injury. He was often sad, and he cried frequently. John disengaged from his family and friends and kept to himself in his bedroom. If he spoke to other people, it was only to apologize for being "useless and worthless." He said he "didn't deserve to live" and would be "better off dead."

John's periods of sadness lasted for two or three weeks at a time. During these episodes, he didn't eat much, slept poorly, and said he was always tired. He tried to go back to work a few times but just couldn't keep up. "I just feel numb," he said. Eventually John's boss had to let him go because his poor performance was endangering the other workers. Once he lost his job, John distanced himself even further from his wife and children, and his wife eventually left him, taking the children with her. Only after his family came apart did John ask his doctor for help, explaining that he had completely lost interest in life and could no longer go on.

The word *depression* has become common in daily conversation. We say we are depressed over a bad relationship, or a bad job situation, or even a bad day. When people use *depression* in this way, they don't mean clinical depression. In general, people use *depression* and *depressed* to describe feeling sad about something that would cause most people to feel sad. If we don't get the promotion we think we deserve, or if we get into a fight with our spouse, or if our child gets into trouble in school, we may call it being depressed, but what we really are feeling is appropriate sadness. Sadness is not pathological. Sadness is a normal human emotion.

Clinical depression, also known as major depression, on the other hand, is a medical diagnosis describing sustained, persistent low (depressed) mood, lasting for many days to weeks, and sometimes even longer, in a person who cannot enjoy usual activities and who may have physical symptoms such as trouble with sleep and concentration.

Unfortunately, inaccurate use of this medical term has permeated popular culture, making it harder for people to understand what depression really is. Our use of the word in this way makes it seem as if depression is not really a medical problem, but rather a "normal" response to life's setbacks. Yet clinical depression is a medical condition and not a normal response to events.

Further complicating the situation is that, even in a medical sense, depression is not a single concept. Depression comes in many forms and has many diagnoses: major depressive disorder, dysthymia, bipolar depression, depressive disorder not otherwise specified, adjustment disorder with depressed mood, and many others. Depression is thus a spectrum of disorders, all of which can affect people mildly or severely, ranging from minor effects on relationships and work to suicide.

What separates a diagnosis of clinical depression from normal sadness—what separates pathology from normality—is whether the symptoms significantly affect functioning. Clinical depression can affect work performance, social relationships, home life, or any combination of these. Furthermore, to warrant the diagnosis of clinical depression, functioning must be persistently affected for a minimum amount of time (two weeks or more for a diagnosis of major depression). Clinical depression is not an afternoon spent mooning around or "having the blues" over a troubling situation. Clinical depression, in fact, can be autonomous, that is, unrelated to any single troubling event. It may occur with no apparent reason and persist for weeks or months. Of course, those who have had a brain injury and their family members may already know from their own experience what major depression is, but using the correct terminology for it affects how people perceive what persons with depression are struggling with.

Symptoms

In brain injury, depressive symptoms are rather common, but in this case we have to be even more careful with terminology, because these symptoms may not fit neatly into a category such as major depressive disorder. Depression in brain injury may be more diffuse and harder to diagnose precisely. Many factors can cause clinical depression after brain injury: having a history of major depression before the injury (a well-known risk factor), the severity of the injury (the more severe, the greater the risk), alcohol or substance abuse, and the presence of psychosocial problems (for example, minimal emotional support, poor finances, unemployment) before and after brain injury. How exactly brain injury causes major depression is unclear. Brain injury can act as a stressor and cause depression in someone who is already vulnerable to depression, or it can cause dysfunction of neural circuits or neurochemicals and trigger depression. Most brain injury researchers believe that it probably does both.

Unfortunately, persons with brain injury or their family members may be told by well-meaning people that it is "understandable" that they are depressed: "Of course you're depressed! Look what you just went through." Even medical professionals may succumb to this fallacy of thinking. But, as we have discussed, it is not normal for a person with brain injury to be depressed—that is, clinically depressed, in the medical sense of the word. Depression is common in brain injury, but it is not necessary. *Clinical depression is not a normal part of recovery from brain injury.*

This is an important distinction. When friends, or family, or even medical personnel accept depression as normal after brain injury, they are doing the person a disservice. The subtle implication is that these symptoms do not deserve treatment; after all, if this depression is normal, why treat it? And what may be implied when depressive symptoms persist is that the person should be "getting over it." So the person with brain injury can interpret this attitude to mean that they have a character flaw or some kind of personal weakness. This message, of course, can make the person feel even worse, thus perpetuating a cycle of deepening depression.

Consider John, in our opening story. His sadness was associated with a number of prolonged, pervasive, and disruptive physical and emotional symptoms. His is a classic example of major depression, also known as clinical depression: a state of persistent sadness or persistent lack of enjoyment often associated with feelings of hopelessness, low self-worth or guilt, and suicidal thoughts. Other symptoms of major depression are changes in sleep, appetite, energy, or concentration, but because these symptoms are also common consequences of the injury to the brain, medical evaluation is necessary to determine whether a person with these symptoms has major depression. Depressive symptoms persist for consecutive days, disrupt the person's life, and interfere with the person's day-to-day functioning. The rate of suicide in people with depression is about 15 percent. Severe major depression can cause hallucinations (hearing, seeing, feeling, or smelling things when there are no external stimuli) or delusions (fixed, false beliefs), or both.

Major depression can interfere with recovery from a brain injury; people with major depression may not recover as well from the brain injury as those without depression, if depression is not treated. Brain injury survivors who suffer from major depression show greater impairment in their ability to function, and they have poorer outcomes than brain injury survivors who are not depressed. Major depression after brain injury can also be associated with alcohol and drug use, which in turn can impair recovery. Alcohol toxicity and brain injury may have a synergistic effect and produce more severe structural brain damage and affect chemical pathways in the brain. Persons with major depressive disorder after brain injury are more likely to be irritable, act aggressively, and be anxious.

Conditions That Mimic Major Depression

We have discussed how major depression is different from normal sadness. However, to complicate matters further, several other disorders may look like major depression but be quite different.

One possibility to consider when a person appears depressed is that the person has bipolar depression. We discuss bipolar disorder in more detail in chapter 12, but we mention it here because depression, along with mania, is part of bipolar disorder. When it's part of bipolar disorder, depression can be hard, even for experts, to distinguish from major depression, but there are some clues. Bipolar depression may begin earlier in life than major depression and have more mood variability and more exaggerated response to stress. The person with bipolar depression may eat more and sleep more (as opposed to eating less and sleeping less, traits more typical in major depression). These are all clues to the possibility of bipolar depression, but the one clear way to distinguish between bipolar depression and major depression is that in bipolar depression, these periods of depression alternate with periods of heightened energy, mood, and activity (mania). The treatment for bipolar depression is quite different from the treatment for major depression, so a correct diagnosis is important.

Another possibility to keep in mind when a person appears depressed is a condition called pseudobulbar affect (PBA), also known as pathological laughing and crying, or emotional incontinence. PBA is fairly common in brain injury, especially in moderate to severe injuries. A person with PBA can cry or laugh for no apparent reason or cry or laugh excessively in relation to what they are reacting to. In other words, someone with PBA may see something on TV that is a bit sad and begin to cry excessively and be unable to stop. Or the person with PBA may not actually feel sad when they are crying; they might be crying for no good reason and not, in truth, be sad at all. The cause of PBA is still not clear. While some believe that it is due to lack of control of emotions due to damage to brain circuits that normally keep emotions in check, others believe that it is related to difficulty with facial expressions, and so crying or laughing can occur without being accompanied by sadness or happiness. Absence of persistent low mood is a key point that differentiates pathological crying of PBA from major depression. Major depression is a mood disorder, and the person suffering from it experiences relentless sadness or lack of enjoyment. In contrast, in pathological crying of PBA, there is tearfulness in the absence of sadness or disproportionately to the sadness felt. Treatment for PBA may be different from treatment for major depression.

Brain Circuits Affected by Major Depression

Clinical depression clearly has a neurobiological basis. We have a fairly good idea at this point what parts of the brain are involved in generating symptoms of depression (figure 11.1). An evolutionarily primitive core area deep within the brain known as the limbic system is involved in generating emotions. The limbic system borders the cortex, the part of the brain involved in thinking and planning.

Parts of the limbic system, including the hippocampus, the amygdala, and the anterior cingulate, are probably involved in the genesis of clinical depression. In fact, current thinking suggests that increased activity in an area of the anterior cingulate called the subgenual cingulate may be associated with depression. The subgenual cingulate is a key part of the neural circuit that connects the frontal lobe cortex (the thinking and planning part of the brain) to the limbic system, the emotional brain. The frontal lobe cortex normally acts as a kind of brake to prevent the subgenual cingulate from getting hyperactive. If this brake fails, the subgenual cingulate is free to become hyperactive, leading to increased emotional discharge—in other words, major depression.

Major depression can occur without directly affecting the limbic system deep within the brain. Damage to the frontal lobe cortex (which, as we've noted, is highly vulnerable to trauma) can result in depression by removing this brake and allowing the limbic system to be hyperactive

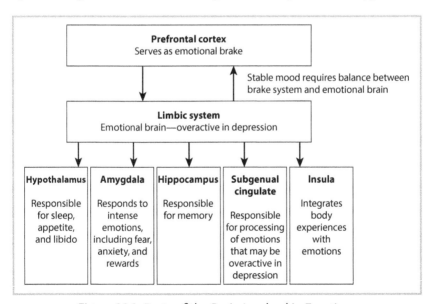

Figure 11.1. Parts of the Brain Involved in Emotions

and letting the "emotional brain" dominate the "thinking and planning brain."

Of course, it is possible for brain trauma to directly affect the limbic system as well, despite its location deep within the brain. The hippocampus portion of the limbic system can shrink in major depression, and shrinkage can be even more pronounced in those who have both brain injury and major depression.

There may be other ways that affecting circuits in the brain, directly or indirectly, leads to major depression. The key concept, however, is that anything that disturbs the balance between the "emotional brain" and the "thinking and planning brain" by making the former more dominant may cause depressive symptoms.

Evidence also suggests that the left frontal cortex in particular is involved in major depression. People who have had left frontal cortex strokes are prone to depression. The left hemisphere of the brain (which houses much of our language abilities) may act as a storyteller of our lives, and this storytelling may decrease the risk of depression. But damage to the left hemisphere may prevent it from creating a story out of life events in an appropriate way, and so may increase the risk of major depression.

Treatment

Treating depression is important because depression itself can have negative biological effects. For instance, research suggests that depression is associated with inflammation in the body. Furthermore, depression can increase the levels of stress hormones such as cortisol or increase adrenaline and impair the immune system. These changes can increase the risk for certain medical illnesses, including heart disease and arthritis. And we know that depression contributes to worse outcomes in people who have had heart attacks or who have diabetes or Alzheimer's disease.

Regardless of the cause, be it the brain injury itself or poor social support, depression has a detrimental effect on the brain. Clinical depression can make patients engage in unsafe behaviors like using drugs or alcohol. People who are clinically depressed may not participate in reha-bilitation as they otherwise would; many ignore their health, eat poorly, and don't exercise.

What can you do if you think you or someone you know and care for is clinically depressed after brain injury? The single most important thing is to get professional help. Only professionals can differentiate among the many faces of depression. Getting an accurate diagnosis from a professional is crucial because treatment differs for different condi-tions. Major depression and similar conditions are often treated with a combination of medication and counseling or psychotherapy.

Medication

Many medications are available to treat depression; all of the standard medications are more or less equally effective but each has different side effects. People with brain injury may be more sensitive than people without brain injury to certain medications. Neuropsychiatrists (doc-tors who are trained in psychiatry and who have experience treating mood, behavioral, and cognitive symptoms in neurologic disorders like brain injury) can choose the most appropriate medications. General psychiatrists, neurologists, physiatrists, and primary care doctors also often treat these symptoms. The medication choice depends on the per-son's emotional and behavioral problems, medical issues, other medica-tions the person is taking, and the person's family medical history. No one should take a medication or adjust the dose of a medication or stop a medication without first getting their doctor's advice.

You may be familiar with the concept that depression is related to a chemical imbalance in the brain resulting from too little serotonin. Serotonin is clearly part of the story of depression. Studies show that people who were depressed and impulsively committed suicide had very low levels of serotonin. Medications for depression, such as selective serotonin reuptake inhibitors (SSRIs), are believed to increase sero-tonin, thus alleviating depression. The success of SSRIs in treating depression has validated the important role of serotonin in depression.

In fact, SSRIs are the mainstay of depression treatment today. Most doctors prefer to treat major depression using SSRIs because of their mild side effects. Common medications in this family include Celexa (citalopram), Zoloft (sertraline), Lexapro (escitalopram), and Prozac (fluoxetine).

The circuitry that we have discussed in this chapter is associated with a significant number of serotonin receptors; there may be a connection between serotonin (part of what we call a chemical model of depression) and the subgenual cingulate (part of a circuitry model of depression).

Other chemicals likely involved in depression are norepinephrine and dopamine. Norepinephrine and dopamine may be important in attention and motivation; many people with depression have problems concentrating and focusing and have trouble getting motivated to do what they know they need to do. Such problems are common after brain injury, and depression can worsen these symptoms. Medications known as selective norepinephrine reuptake inhibitors (SNRIs) increase norepinephrine and serotonin levels and help depression. Examples of SNRIs are medications like Effexor (venlafaxine), Pristiq (desvenlafaxine), and Fetzima (levomilnacipran). Wellbutrin (bupropion) increases dopamine levels predominantly.

The chemical and circuitry models are likely both correct; they just explain depression at two different levels. But things may be more complicated than that. Despite their names, SSRIs and SNRIs don't simply increase serotonin and alleviate depression. If they did, SSRIs and SNRIs would work very quickly, within hours or days. They don't. They take weeks to work, and here's why: SSRIs and other antidepressants stimulate physical remodeling of the brain. That is, they cause brain circuits to grow and change, using the brain's power of neural plasticity. This process takes weeks, and the mechanism of remodeling, which takes time, explains the few weeks' lag between when a person begins taking antidepressants and when they feel their full effects.

This remodeling process ties in with our earlier discussion of inflammation. Levels of certain chemicals called growth factors may increase when a person is taking SSRIs. These increased growth factor levels stimulate growth in brain circuits. Inflammation may impair these growth factors, and so impair brain remodeling

In discussing neuronal circuits and neurochemistry we do not mean to suggest that there is no psychosocial component to depression. There certainly is. Clearly, poor support from family, an unstable living situation, or a stressful work environment can worsen mood in people who have depression. These psychosocial factors, however, also work by means of some of the same mechanisms in the brain as the brain injury itself. That is, psychosocial factors may worsen depression by affecting some of the same circuits, via serotonin and/or other brain chemicals, and by affecting growth factors. They may cause emotional hyperreactivity in the limbic system. They may cause "faulty thoughts" in the frontal cortex, allowing the emotional brain to dominate behavior.

In other words, some people are particularly vulnerable to life stressors because they have abnormal levels of serotonin, norepinephrine, or dopamine. When they have a major life stressor such as a brain injury, they are prone to an increase in inflammatory chemicals, which can lead to an increase of cortisol, a stress hormone. This increase in cortisol can lead to shrinkage of the hippocampus and to an imbalance between the emotional brain and the thinking brain. The thinking brain cannot curb the overactive emotional brain, and the result is emotional instability. This is one model of how to think about depression; however, scientists are still in the process of studying and understanding the different biological, psychological, and environmental factors and their interactions in the development of clinical depression.

It is important to clarify that SSRIs are a suitable treatment for major depression. But the treatment for bipolar depression is quite different, and in fact, if someone has bipolar disorder and is put on an SSRI only, there is the possibility that symptoms overall could get worse. Bipolar disorder often needs a mood stabilizer like Depakote (valproic acid), Lithobid or Eskalith (lithium), Lamictal (lamotrigine), or Tegretol (carbamazepine). Oftentimes, another agent is necessary. Seroquel (quetiapine), Vraylar (cariprazine), and Latuda (lurasidone) are approved by the FDA for acute treatment of bipolar depression.

Pseudobulbar affect (PBA) may potentially be treated with SSRI medications. Nuedexta (dextromethorphan/quinidine) is a medication approved by the FDA for treating PBA in neurological conditions, with evidence from multiple sclerosis and amyotrophic lateral sclerosis (ALS, or Lou Gehrig's disease). Nuedexta specifically reduces the symptoms of PBA only; it does not treat depression. It is not yet entirely clear if PBA symptoms in brain injury would respond to Nuedexta in the same way as PBA symptoms in multiple sclerosis or ALS.

Neuromodulation Therapy

Neuromodulation therapy alters or modulates parts of the brain directly using forces such as electricity or magnetism. Repeated application of these forces to parts of the brain over time can cause changes in the way neurons in those parts of the brain interact. The importance of appreciating brain circuitry is that new neuromodulation techniques for treating clinical depression may directly or indirectly affect parts of the brain circuits associated with depression.

Transcranial magnetic stimulation (TMS) is a technique that uses an electromagnetic coil, placed over the scalp, focused on the left prefrontal cortex, which as we have discussed, plays a major role in depression. The coil generates brief magnetic pulses, which pass through the bony skull and into the brain and stimulate neurons to fire. The concept is that "neurons that fire together wire together." As neurons in the prefrontal cortex fire more due to magnetic stimulation, more connections are made between them. As more connections are made, the prefrontal cortex can be more effective (much like building up connections through road networks can make transit more effective). TMS directly enhances neural plasticity and helps the prefrontal cortex "tune and prune" its connections in a favorable way.

Activating the frontal cortex with this technology does ameliorate depression; TMS is an FDA-cleared treatment for major depression in the general population. Ongoing studies are working to determine the effectiveness of TMS in persons with brain injury and depression.

Additional treatment techniques currently under study are magnetic seizure therapy, in which a magnetic field is used to induce seizures that may help depression, and transient direct current stimulation, in which a weak electrical current is applied to the brain.

Electroconvulsive therapy (ECT), or "shock therapy," is another neuromodulation technique. While the treatment has been around for decades, improvements over the years have made it more tolerable and more focused. In fact, today ECT is a treatment of choice for severe depression. Research studies suggest that most persons who have received ECT may have memory loss for events that occur around the time ECT was administered, but the memory loss can sometimes go back for months. However, memory usually returns in a few months after ECT. Our clinical experience and available research suggest that ECT is safe and effective in people with brain injury. As far as is known, the pattern of memory loss is similar to that in people without brain injury.

Deep brain stimulation (DBS), a research tool currently, involves placing electrodes within certain areas of the brain to produce electrical impulses that can regulate brain chemicals or abnormal electrical activity within the brain. For the treatment of major depression, electrodes are implanted in the subgenual cingulate, among other regions of the brain. When activated, these electrodes act as a kind of pacemaker for the brain, activating the frontal cortex and deactivating the subgenual cingulate.

Psychedelics

Psychedelic (and similar) medications are an exciting new possibility to treat depression. They work more directly, more quickly, and more effectively than traditional antidepressants by enhancing neural plasticity. Ketamine is an example of such a medication, as it has psychedelic effects, though it is not technically a psychedelic pharmacologically. It has long been used as a sedative and anesthetic, but at low doses it can help with depression as well. One of the ways that ketamine works is by blocking glutamate N-Methyl-D-aspartate (NMDA) receptors on inhibitory neurons in the prefrontal cortex. Glutamate is a neurotransmitter that is fast-acting and critical for much of the brain's functioning. In fact, glutamate (and its derivative, GABA) are much more common than any of the neurotransmitters that we have discussed so far, such as serotonin. Glutamate is important for neural firing, and blocking of glutamate receptors can decrease neural firing. Ketamine, by blocking firing of inhibitory neurons in the prefrontal cortex, may actually stimulate firing of neurons in this part of the brain overall. You can think about this like "a negative of a negative is a positive." As we have seen, increased firing of neurons in the prefrontal cortex enhances neural plasticity and improves functioning of this critical part of the brain.

Studies have shown ketamine to be a rapid-acting antidepressant. A single low, sub-anesthetic dose of ketamine given as an infusion through the veins may help to relieve depression within a few hours. However, ketamine has not been FDA-approved for the treatment of depression. But its component, esketamine, given as a nasal spray, has been FDA-approved for treatment-resistant depression. There are limited studies of its use in the general population and details such as its safety, duration of treatment, and dosing are still being worked out. Esketamine and ketamine are also not without side effects; common ones include dissociation, sedation, and potential for abuse. At this time, there is limited research on the use of ketamine or esketamine in the brain injury population.

Other psychedelics such as psylocibin and MDMA (commonly known as Ecstasy or Molly) are currently being studied for the treatment of major depression and other disorders such as PTSD in the general population. From results so far from research studies, psylocibin may also more quickly and more effectively improve depression than standard antidepressants. Again, we have limited information yet on applicability to persons with brain injury.

Psychotherapy

Psychotherapy (or talk therapy) is a form of treatment that aims to teach skills and approaches to better understand and manage emotional reactions, as we discussed in chapter 7. Psychotherapy offers techniques for coping with stressful circumstances and negative thoughts. All forms of depression respond well to psychotherapy in combination with appropriate antidepressant medications (when needed). A mental health professional can choose the type and the duration of psychotherapy that is best for each person. Psychologists (who have PhD degrees), mental health therapists, and clinical social workers (who have LCSW certification or MSW degrees) can do therapy. Most forms of talk therapy are short-term, focused, and specific in their approach.

Supportive Therapy

The goal of supportive therapy is to provide hope and to educate about the illness or the circumstances associated with stress and depression. Supportive therapy in the case of brain injury could include discussing how the injury has affected the person's outlook and family. The therapist can provide concrete suggestions about how best to adjust to the new life situation the person is facing.

Cognitive Behavioral Therapy

Cognitive behavioral therapy (CBT) is based on the principle that thoughts and feelings influence a person's behavior. Thoughts can lead to certain feelings, which in turn can lead to behaviors (figure 11.2). The concept of CBT is to train someone to think more like a scientist, to examine whether the thoughts they are having are valid or supported by evidence. A person who has depression may have thoughts pop into their mind that are not supported by evidence (for example, "I will never get better" or "It's no use" or "No one likes me"). In CBT, the person learns not to accept any thoughts that come into their mind without examining them and being skeptical of their validity.

Therapists trained in CBT teach the person they are working with to recognize negative thought patterns and to substitute more realistic ones for the negative ones. In this way, the person's behavior can be converted to more productive and healthy activities. CBT therapists usually see the person once a week for a set period of time (for example, 12 weeks). At the end of each session, the therapist may assign homework so that the person continues to practice working with their thoughts every day as they go about their life. CBT can also be simply behavior therapy or behavior modification therapy (the behavioral aspect of CBT), the goal being to change abnormal behavior and to help the person unlearn behavior patterns that contribute to their feelings of sadness or make them worse. Behavioral therapies provided by experienced professionals also include relaxation training (training to attain a sense of calmness and reduce tension), stress management (training to identify stressors and learn healthy coping skills), biofeedback (training to control various body function using electronic or other instruments), exposure therapy (exposing the person to the situation that triggers anxiety or fear but done by an experienced professional in a safe setting), desensitization (a type of gradual exposure therapy), and mindfulness meditation (a type of stress reduction therapy focused on being present with the here and now and accepting one's thoughts and feelings without judging or berating themselves).

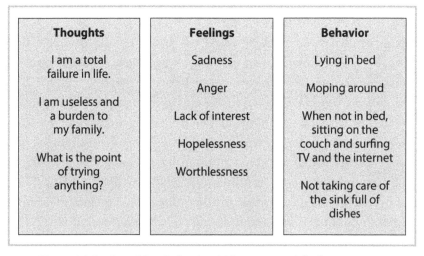

Thoughts	Feelings	Behavior
I am a total failure in life.	Sadness	Lying in bed
	Anger	Moping around
I am useless and a burden to my family.	Lack of interest	When not in bed, sitting on the couch and surfing TV and the internet
	Hopelessness	
What is the point of trying anything?	Worthlessness	Not taking care of the sink full of dishes

Figure 11.2. Cognitive Behavioral Therapy Model of Depression

Acceptance and Commitment Therapy

This is a type of cognitive and behavioral therapy which focuses on helping the person accept their thoughts and emotions, being in the present, not being judgmental, and learning and making a commitment to live in accordance with their values and goals.

Interpersonal Therapy

Personal interactions can be problematic because of the physical and emotional consequences of brain injury; clinical depression on top of those conditions can lead to poor communication and an inability to express emotion. The goal of interpersonal therapy (IPT) is to help the person improve interpersonal skills and either resolve or cope with interpersonal problems. IPT focuses on learning effective communication, expressing emotions appropriately, and being appropriately assertive (that is, learning which situations call for assertiveness and how to be assertive when appropriate). IPT can help the person with a brain injury regain or improve these communication skills.

Dialectical Behavioral Therapy

Dialectical behavioral therapy (DBT) focuses on distressing problematic behaviors and helps the person learn different, more rewarding approaches. The therapist usually focuses on one problematic event at a time and works with the person to understand the events that triggered the behavior. DBT incorporates mindfulness (keeping the mind in the present and accepting one's thoughts and emotions in a nonjudgmental way), a technique often used in cognitive behavioral therapy. DBT teaches skills for regulating emotions and not overreacting to people or events. DBT can be particularly helpful for people who may be overwhelmed by emotions and consider harming themselves.

Family Therapy

Family therapy is helpful for people with brain injury, and we strongly urge families who are finding it difficult to adjust and cope after their loved one's brain injury to incorporate it. The family therapist brings together all the family members who are willing to participate in therapy, educates them about brain injury and its consequences, encourages them to acknowledge and talk about the stress in the family (and their relationship with the brain-injured person), and offers strategies to reduce the stress and cope with all the issues raised. Family therapy can incorporate techniques from supportive and cognitive behavioral therapy as well.

Group Therapy

In group therapy a small number of people with similar issues meet regularly (often weekly) with a therapist to discuss their problems and discuss ways of dealing with them. The goal is for patients to learn from one another, with the benefit of professional guidance and feedback from the therapist. It can be hard for people with brain injury to find others who understand what they have gone through, what they are feeling now, and the anxieties they have about the future. Sharing concerns, fears, small victories, and coping techniques with others who have experienced similar trauma can be beneficial to people with brain injury.

In summary, major depression that develops after brain injury can be a serious impediment to recovery; it should not be minimized or normalized. If you experience symptoms of major depression or notice them in a family member you care for, take quick action to get help. Major depression after brain injury can result directly from the brain injury itself or indirectly from other factors such as loss of a job, trauma related to the injury, or unsupportive family. Major depression can make symptoms of the brain injury worse, cause recovery to falter, and contribute to other medical problems. It can be a fatal illness. Suicide is not uncommon in people who have major depression. We ignore it at our own and our loved one's peril. If you don't know where to get started in helping yourself or your family member suffering from depression and suicidal thoughts, call your primary care doctor, neurologist, or other trusted professional for suggestions and referrals. If you are unable to find a physician, you can also contact your state or national brain injury associations for help regarding finding a provider or any questions you may have regarding the brain injury.

If you are concerned about the safety of your family member or friend call 911 or take them to the nearest hospital. Self-injurious behavior is not uncommon in depression. Take seriously any comments they may make about suicide and obtain professional help for them. The National Suicide Prevention Lifeline provides free counseling and support for people in distress 24–7. The phone number is 988.

Tips and tools on how to manage the symptoms discussed in this chapter are available in tables 11.1 and 11.2.

TABLE 11.1. TIPS AND TOOLS FOR COPING WITH DEPRESSION AFTER BRAIN INJURY

Get Help	Depression in any form is treatable.
	Get help from a mental health professional.
	Avoid self-diagnosing.
	Avoid self-treating with alcohol/illicit drugs.
	Never give up: medications and therapy take time to work.
	Ask your health care professional about other treatment strategies if your current strategy is not working.
A Healthy Body = A Healthy Brain	Maintaining a healthy lifestyle is an important aspect of management.
	Exercise regularly—try for 30 minutes a day (even broken down over multiple periods) three to four times per week. Exercise helps with both physical and mental recovery.
	Practice sleep hygiene—go to bed and wake up around the same time every day; use your bed only for sleep and physical intimacy; avoid caffeinated drinks after 2 p.m.; keep the bedroom quiet, dim, and relaxing.

Table 11.1 continued on next page

Maintain Consistency	Consistency is key to recovery—whether it is taking your medications, exercising, eating healthy, or maintaining a routine.
	The brain tends to respond well to structure and organization, which may assist with both physical and emotional recovery.
	Make healthy habits your default.
Stay Organized; Stay Busy	Keep your brain active just by going about your day-to-day activities, such as conversing with others, completing chores, and engaging in your usual pleasurable activities.
	Talk to your clinician about referral to an occupational therapist, who can help with structuring the day.
	Learn new puzzles, games, or crafts, all of which have the potential to enhance neuroplasticity.
Keep It Simple	Keep it simple and start with what you enjoy most.
	As you feel comfortable, gradually step up your activities to include tasks that are more challenging.
	Build in rest breaks; do not "push through" fatigue.
	Use your own body as a barometer to recognize and measure the signs of fatigue.
Say No to Alcohol and Drugs	Avoid using alcohol and illicit drugs.
	Continued use of alcohol and other mind-altering drugs can worsen mood states, so people with brain injury and depression need to abstain from their use as much as possible.
	If you find that you cannot stop using alcohol or drugs on your own, seek professional help.

TABLE 11.2. TIPS AND TOOLS FOR CARING FOR SOMEONE WITH DEPRESSION AFTER BRAIN INJURY

Emphasize Safety	If you are concerned about the safety of the person you are caring for, call 911 or take them to the nearest hospital.
	Self-injurious behavior is not uncommon in persons with major depression.
	Take seriously any comments they may make about suicide and obtain professional help for them.
Offer Loving Care	Offer support and understanding.
	Major depression is not a sign of weakness or a character flaw.
	Your consistent support and understanding are valuable to the person recovering from brain injury.
Encourage Engagement	Social withdrawal and isolation are common in people with major depression.
	Encourage and even join the person with brain injury in participating in fun activities, hobbies, and connecting with family and friends.
Balance Independence versus Dependence	Balance too much versus too little involvement.
	People with major depression may appear hostile and angry and reject your attempts to provide care; conversely, they can become very dependent on you and shadow you everywhere.
	Find a middle ground.
	Encourage the person with brain injury to make decisions, but if they get stuck, offer choices.

Table 11.2 continued on next page

You Are Not a Machine	You cannot go on and on, 24-7.
	Take care of yourself.
	Do not hesitate to obtain professional help if you're feelng stressed or overwhelmed.
	Do not be harsh or critical of yourself.
	You cannot be 100 percent always.
	Remember there are things you cannot always control.
Find a Support Network	Contact your state's Brain Injury Association regarding support groups in your area.
	Do not isolate yourself; do not be shy about getting assistance; asking for help and finding other resources is a strength, not a weakness.
Taking Care of Yourself Is a Virtue, Not a Vice	Take time off to relax and have fun.
	Eat healthy meals.
	Make time to exercise or do other enjoyable activities.
	Do not overload your schedule.
	Make sure the activities you have set for yourself or your loved one are doable and attainable.
	Do not feel guilty about taking care of yourself.
	You cannot be in a fight-or-flight response all the time.

Take-Home Points

Major depression is not uncommon after a brain injury, and there are many treatment options to help address it.

Major depression is a treatable illness.

Treatment of major depression is often multimodal and includes a combination of therapies with or without medication.

The National Suicide Prevention Lifeline provides free counseling and support for people in distress 24-7. The phone number is 988.

Connect with the state or national brain injury associations for any
questions you may have regarding the brain injury.

Exercise

*Here is a simple exercise to identify unhelpful thought patterns
and replace them with more helpful ones. Let's use an example:
Perhaps you have been thinking about the recent loss of your job,
which makes you feel like "a complete failure." You feel frustrated
and hopeless. To address these feelings, follow these steps:*

• *First, write down what your thoughts are and how they make
you feel.*

• *Next, take a few minutes to examine the thoughts. Ask yourself,
"What evidence do I have that I am a complete failure?"*

• *Next, really examine how the thoughts make you feel. Notice
how much thinking about them makes you feel more and more
frustrated.*

• *Now, see if you can change the automatic thought you have
developed. For example, "I was not able to keep my job after the
injury, because it is just a lot harder to get things done. I have
been doing well in helping around the house more with chores.
Maybe I could spend more time helping to take care of household
chores and consider a part-time job at some point."*

• *Finally, think about what your behavior is when you have these
thoughts and feelings. Do you disengage and watch television?
Do you become irritable and confrontational with your family?
Changing your behavior can really help change your emotions
and shift your thoughts. For example, "Every time I think about
losing my job, I really don't feel like doing anything at all so I spend
the day watching television." Instead of the automatic behavior,
decide to go for a walk every time you have these thoughts.*

• *Sometimes it can be helpful to rate your mood to see what is most helpful. For example, before doing the exercise, ask yourself, on a scale of 0–10, how frustrated do I feel? Then do the exercise. Then rate your frustration again on a scale on 0–10. However, don't worry if your mood doesn't improve drastically. These things take time. Also, some people find it helpful to rate their mood, while others become too focused on the number— which causes additional distress. Do what works best for you as an individual.*

Chapter 12

Mania

Darlene suffered a right brain stroke at age 65, which required a short period of hospitalization in a stroke unit followed by extensive rehabilitation. Darlene had no personal psychiatric illness prior to the stroke but did have a strong family history of bipolar disorder in two of her younger siblings and her paternal aunt. Her physical symptoms gradually improved, and she remained physically and emotionally stable for about a year.

Then her husband noticed that from time to time Darlene was extremely cheerful. She talked very fast, switching from one topic to another, and seemed to have endless energy, yet slept only one or two hours a night: "I don't know what happens to her sometimes. It's like she's on speed—she just goes on and on and *on*." Her husband also noticed that she was acting in ways she had never done before the stroke. She was quick to anger and cursed often. Darlene also started spending lavishly on things she did not need—expensive perfumes, clothes, shoes, handbags, and high-end jewelry. These periods would last for about a week to ten days, and then her mood would slowly return to normal. She wasn't irritable or agitated, and she rarely got upset over anything—she was back to the "old" Darlene. Her mood would be even-keeled, with enough energy to do normal chores and sleep at night for about seven to eight hours.

Two years after the stroke, however, during another episode, Darlene became so energized and grandiose with beliefs that she was a superwoman that she came close to jumping out the attic window. Her husband stopped her just in time and called her doctor, who admitted Darlene to an acute-care psychiatric facility. Her husband told the admitting staff that Darlene had experienced several such episodes, but of milder severity, over the two years since the stroke. These episodes were similar to some of the episodes her brother, who had symptoms consistent with bipolar I disorder, had experienced, he told them, but he insisted that Darlene had never exhibited these symptoms before her stroke.

Darlene stayed in the hospital for about two weeks and was treated with both an antipsychotic, Seroquel (quetiapine), and a mood stabilizer, Depakote (valproic acid). She responded very well to the combined medications and was discharged to an outpatient facility with recommendations for regular follow-up.

One of the emotional disorders that can occur after traumatic brain injury is mania, a state of heightened mental and physical activity. Everything about the person with mania is sped up—elated mood, excess energy, racing thoughts, and almost frantic activity.

Some people might wonder why mania is considered a problem. After all, most of us probably wouldn't mind some extra energy, and the feeling of euphoria seems desirable. Unfortunately, along with the increased energy and euphoria, other symptoms of mania, such as impulsivity and reckless behaviors, can cause problems, as when Darlene came close to jumping out the window.

Symptoms

Classic symptoms of mania are exaggerated or irritable mood, decreased need for sleep (for days), racing thoughts, grandiose thoughts, rapid-fire speech that is hard to interrupt, restlessness, and impulsivity. It's common for people in a manic state to go for days without sleeping or sleep only for a few hours a night. They initiate many tasks at once yet fail to complete any of them, and they can exhibit abnormal behavior, such as spending sprees or an overactive sex drive. Aggression, edginess, hallucinations, and delusions are also common symptoms of mania, symptoms that may get out of control, interfere with day-to-day activities, and require hospitalization.

In the person with brain injury, these manifestations of mania may be intermittent and episodic, but some symptoms, such as irritability, mild aggression, and impulsivity, may persist and become part of the person's new baseline personality. The medical diagnosis in such cases is "personality change secondary to traumatic brain injury." When treating a person with these symptoms, clinicians may call family members to find out if the heightened state of activity is persistent or intermittent.

Darlene, because she had normal mood states between her episodes, with no irritability, agitation, or aggression, was suffering only from mania, not a permanent personality change. The person with brain injury should be evaluated as soon as possible for these aggressive behaviors, because hyperexcitability and impulsivity can lead to reckless and dangerous behavior (such as jumping out a window).

Mania, or a milder version called hypomania, can combine with personality changes due to brain injury. Mania is time limited—lasting days to weeks—but personality change secondary to TBI is more persistent and may be permanent.

Mania can occur as part of bipolar (previously known as manic-depressive) illness not related to brain injury, since bipolar disorder is predominantly a genetically based illness. In bipolar I, a manic phase alternates with major depression. Bipolar II is a variant characterized by major depressive episodes alternating with hypomania. It is also possible to have mixed features, where a predominant state of mood (depression, mania, or hypomania) also has several symptoms of the opposite polarity (figure 12.1). Mania that develops after a brain injury can look the same as the mania of bipolar disorder.

Research suggests that mania, even though not common after brain injury, can develop in people with injuries to the frontal and temporal lobes. We know that brain shrinkage and damage to the prefrontal cortex, amygdala, and basal ganglia can also cause mania. Dysfunction

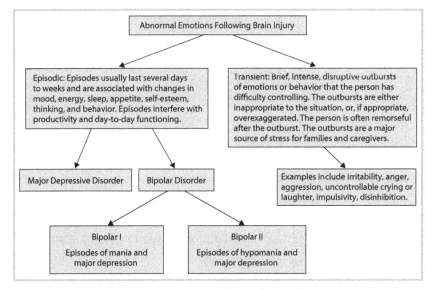

Figure 12.1. Types of Mood Disorders

with the brain chemicals serotonin, dopamine, and norepinephrine may also be associated with bipolar disorder. Some researchers suggest a "double-hit" theory: that is, manic episodes occur after brain injury in those who already have some predisposing factors, such as a family history of bipolar disorder.

Treatment

Acute worsening of mood or sudden change in mood in a person with brain injury needs immediate medical evaluation. In many cases, the person with brain injury may not recognize that their symptoms are worsening. Family members should contact the person's doctor immediately; if the doctor cannot be reached, the family should take the person to be evaluated in the closest emergency department. If the person is very agitated or aggressive and the family is unable to contact the doctor, they should call 911. They can even request the dispatcher to send the mobile crisis team or the crisis intervention team (CIT) officer on duty.

Sudden, unexplained changes in mood require immediate treatment with medications; mood stabilizers and antipsychotics are typical treatments for mania. Common mood stabilizers are lithium, Depakote (valproic acid), Lamictal (lamotrigine), and Tegretol (carbamazepine). Seroquel (quetiapine), Risperdal (risperidone), and Zyprexa (olanzapine) are examples of antipsychotics.

After mood stabilization, it is important for the person to continue outpatient treatment, as Darlene did, focusing on monitoring signs and symptoms, observing medication compliance, and adjusting medications as needed. Some of these medications require the patient to have regular blood work done to check the drug levels in the blood, since low doses may not be effective, and high doses can be toxic.

It is best for the person with brain injury–induced mania to abstain from using alcohol and illicit drugs. Mood-altering substances can make the symptoms of mania worse, particularly impulsivity, and impulsivity prompts risky behaviors.

Behavioral and talk therapy can be helpful in combination with medication. Supportive therapy focuses on educating the person about brain injury and mood symptoms (in both the early and later stages of the diagnosis) and offers healthy strategies to prevent or minimize stress, since stress can be a trigger for a manic episode.

In summary, untreated mania/hypomania is a potentially dangerous condition, because people with mania have minimal insight into their illness and may indulge in risky and life-threatening behaviors. As a family member or caregiver helping the person with brain injury experiencing mania, seeking professional treatment and ensuring they remain engaged in treatment will go a long way in preventing or at least minimizing manic episodes. Stressors can worsen episodes of mania, so reduce stress as much as possible and work with them to handle stress. If you notice early signs of relapse—sleeping less than usual, becoming more irritable or euphoric for no particular reason, or excessive energy and activity—encourage them to see their doctor.

Tips and tools on how to manage the symptoms discussed in this chapter appear in tables 12.1 and 12.2.

TABLE 12.1. TIPS AND TOOLS FOR COPING WITH MANIA AFTER BRAIN INJURY

Adhere to Treatment	Do not adjust or stop medications without first consulting your doctor. Do not take extra doses if you miss taking your medicine (unless specifically ordered by your doctor or health care provider). Medications can be extremely helpful in managing mania. Stick to treatment even after the manic crisis resolves.
Develop a Safety Plan	Anticipate crises and have an emergency action plan including: • Contact information for doctors • Medication list including dosages • List of medical problems • Medication allergies • Contact information for people your doctors can talk to • List of medications that you've tried before—this information will make your doctor more efficient
Say No to Alcohol and Drugs	People with mania after brain injury should abstain from using alcohol and illicit drugs. Continued use of alcohol and other mind-altering drugs can worsen mood states. If you find that you cannot stop using alcohol or drugs on your own, seek professional help.
Stick to Routine	Maintain a routine, including a sleep schedule. Avoid shift work when possible, as changing between day and night shifts can affect mood.

TABLE 12.2. TIPS AND TOOLS FOR CARING FOR SOMEONE EXPERIENCING MANIA AFTER BRAIN INJURY	
Emphasize Safety	Call 911 or take the individual to the hospital if you are concerned about safety.
	Safety comes first and trumps all other issues: someone in a manic episode may be agitated or even aggressive.
	When you call 911, ask the dispatcher to send the mobile crisis team or the officer on duty for the crisis intervention team, if available.
Consult If Concerned	Seek medical help as soon as possible if you notice a sudden change in the person's mood and behavior.
	To work with a psychiatrist, ideally a neuropsychiatrist who has training in both brain injury and psychiatric symptoms, is very important in the context of mania and associated disorders.
Collaborate, Don't Confront	Asking the person what would be helpful and what they are experiencing is a good place to start.
	The person who is going through a manic phase may have limited or no awareness of their problem and may refuse treatment, so you need to be careful— gentle but firm.
Minimize and Manage Stress	Be aware that excessive or unmanaged stress can trigger a manic episode.
	Learn what triggers manic episodes (such as stopping or reducing medication without consulting their doctor or using alcohol, marijuana, or other drugs), and help the person reduce or avoid these stressors.

Table 12.2 continued on next page

Listen, Learn, and Negotiate	Practice active-listening skills.
	Ask open-ended questions encouraging the person to share concerns that can lead to solutions.
	For example, if the person insists on not taking their medication, ask them to tell you a bit about that decision; if they say the medicine is causing drowsiness, consult with the doctor about moving it to nighttime or reducing the dose.

Take-Home Points

Mania is not just a state of being overjoyed or very happy. It is a heightened state of mood, energy, and activity that can be lethal if not treated medically.

Collaboration with a psychiatrist can be extremely helpful in managing mania/hypomania following brain injury.

Maintain a safety plan and keep it handy.

Exercise

• Maintain a simple mood log. Every day (around the same time), write down a few words to describe your mood. This information can help your doctor understand if medications are helping to manage symptoms.

• Complete a safety plan. Enlist two or three people you trust who can help you to stay grounded. Conduct "reality checks" with them if you notice changes in your mood or behavior. If so, have them contact your doctor for help.

• Make a list of things to do and things to avoid to stay balanced.

Chapter 13

Anxiety

Sara was 43 when she was involved in a serious car accident that resulted in bleeding within her brain. She did well and made gradual progress throughout much of her prolonged hospitalization and eventual rehabilitation. After Sara returned home, however, her husband noticed that she was becoming more and more anxious. She worried excessively about everyday matters. For example, she worried about their children taking the school bus; her concern lasted until they came home. Later in the day, she worried about having dinner ready at the scheduled time or going to bed at her usual time. Her husband also noticed that she worried chronically for no apparent reason about minor things—"this, that, and the other," as he called it. He worried aloud that "she's become a nervous wreck." In addition, Sara was easily distracted, was having trouble falling asleep, and complained of being tired during the day. At first, her husband brushed off these changes as worries related to her accident and hospitalization. But when Sara's anxiety was still problematic after nine months and continued to interfere with her day-to-day functioning, her husband decided to get professional help.

Anxiety is common after brain injury and can often occur along with depression. Of course, everyone gets anxious to some degree. In fact, there is a very good reason for our brains to have circuits for anxiety: anxiety helps us avoid danger. Without anxiety we would be much more likely to put ourselves in danger, and once in danger, not get away quickly enough. Without anxiety, our ancestors would have been regular meals for saber-toothed tigers, as they would not have had the sense to get away from these predators.

The anxiety circuits in the brain probably developed as threat detectors. They allow us to scan the environment for threats, and they motivate us to escape from these threats and avoid them in the future. These anxiety circuits, like any other parts of the brain, can sustain damage in a brain injury, and when they are damaged, patients can develop excess anxiety to the point that it interferes with treatment in the hospital, in rehabilitation, or in their ability to adjust to their normal routines after returning home. These symptoms can create additional friction when family and friends do not realize that the anxiety stems from brain damage.

One of the key parts of the brain involved in anxiety generation is the amygdala, deep within the brain, around the level of the temples. The amygdala senses danger and is part of the memory system of the brain. It is particularly good at remembering threats and is activated when there is a possible threat. When the amygdala senses a threat, it activates other parts of the brain, including the hypothalamus (figure 13.1). The hypothalamus in turn activates the fight-or-flight mechanism by releasing hormones like cortisol-releasing factor (CRF). CRF acts on the pituitary gland, and adrenocorticotropic hormone (ACTH) is released, which in turn acts on the adrenal glands, situated above the kidneys. The adrenal glands release norepinephrine (also known as noradrenaline), which prepares the body to "fight" or "flee." Blood pressure and blood sugar rise, increasing the supply of energy in the arms and legs to deal with the situation. The heart rate accelerates and breathing rate increases. Combined, all these physical changes can fuel a subjective sense of anxiety.

Damage to anxiety circuits can change people's personalities—instead of becoming more anxious, they might become more impulsive, more risk-prone, and less anxious in situations that they would have avoided before. They can become very different people from who they were before the injury. These personality changes can cause addition-

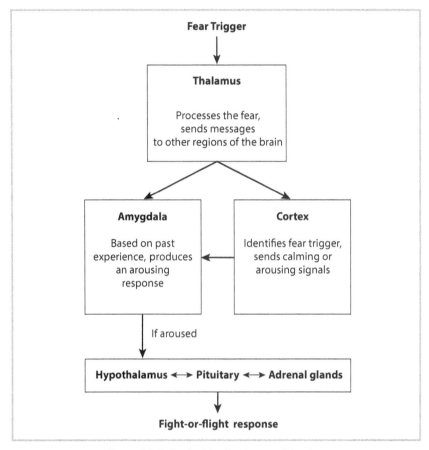

Figure 13.1. Brain Mechanisms of Anxiety

al problems during treatment and after returning home. Family and friends may not understand why their loved one is so different now, leading to misery on both sides.

Symptoms

Anxiety comes in various forms. Some people with brain injury have persistent free-floating anxiety for prolonged periods that interferes with their everyday activities. The medical term for this condition is *generalized anxiety disorder* (GAD). The anxiety symptoms Sara experienced are consistent with GAD. In addition to chronic worry, people with GAD are more on edge and look for danger when there are no obvious reasons for concern. In a sense, their anxiety circuits are overactive. They are perpetually scanning the environment for potential danger. It's like they're looking for the saber-toothed tigers on the plain when, in reality, there are none. Everyday stresses and strains of life affect people with GAD more than the general population. People with this activated anxiety tend to be more irritable, have trouble with sleep, complain of muscle tension, and feel fatigued. They may realize that they are having trouble controlling how much they worry. It can be difficult for family and friends to interact as before with people who develop generalized anxiety disorder after brain injury.

If you are involved in the care of a person with brain injury who has been suffering from anxiety after the injury, keep in mind that they are not purposely being difficult; being excessively anxious can certainly come out as irritability and impatience, but such behavior doesn't mean that they are targeting you.

Pronounced anxiety can trigger panic attacks—sudden waves of anxiety that occur without warning. A panic attack can be so severe that the person experiencing it sometimes feels that they are about to die. Classic symptoms of a panic attack are racing heartbeat, shortness of breath, and a feeling of impending doom. A panic attack is an intense experience that often leads to emergency department visits. Panic attacks can be more prevalent in some people after a brain injury, especially if they were prone to them beforehand.

Anxiety can lead to agitation in some people, especially if they have periods of confusion. This confusion, especially immediately after a severe brain injury, is called delirium, an altered state of consciousness somewhere between being awake and being asleep. People experiencing delirium can see things that are not really there (hallucinations) or believe that people, even their doctors or family and friends, are trying to hurt them. In defending themselves against these perceived threats, they can become physically aggressive or agitated. This behavior can be disturbing to family members, who may not understand why their loved one is frightened of them or fighting them. In the hospital, people with delirium may require sedation or, rarely, physical restraint. As disturbing as this can be to family and caregivers, these periods of confusion and high anxiety are temporary. As the brain recovers from the injury, confusion lessens, and the anxiety abates.

Anxiety can also manifest as agitation, irritability, frustration, or outbursts of anger in people with brain injury who cannot adequately express their emotions. Such bouts of anxiety are usually triggered by actual or perceived stressful situations. For example, simple activities of daily living such as bathing and dressing may be a source of stress and anxiety in persons with severe brain injury for a number of reasons: embarrassment about their loss of independence, guilt about having to depend on their loved ones, or resentment that someone is invading their privacy. Anxiety can manifest as frustration or irritability even in those with mild to moderate brain injury, when they encounter situations that they could easily have managed before the injury, such as maintaining accounts or planning an event. They may not verbalize their anxiety but express it physically in a flushing face, pacing, fidgeting, muttering, or even screaming.

In some people, anxiety can manifest primarily as general physical symptoms; especially after brain injury, whose common aftereffects include dizziness and headaches, it can be difficult to differentiate between what is due to anxiety and what is due to the direct effects of the brain injury. In many cases, the two causes coexist: dizziness may come from the brain injury but may persist because of the anxiety.

Post-traumatic stress disorder (PTSD) has historically been thought of as an anxiety disorder (though thinking about its role as an anxiety disorder is changing) that develops after exposure to a stressful and traumatic event. PTSD can start weeks or months after exposure to the event and last anywhere from a few weeks to several months. During this time, the person reexperiences the trauma in flashbacks or dreams. The person is vigilant and tends to avoid people, places, or situations associated with the traumatic event. With brain injury, especially mild brain injury, PTSD can co-occur with the brain injury. Soldiers stunned by shrapnel from explosive devices can lose consciousness momentarily and have trouble with memory for several hours, but they may also struggle with mental images of the explosion, the screams of civilians, the smell of sulfur and burning flesh, and guilt about others in their unit dying. These repetitive images, thoughts, and anxieties may become chronic and haunt them for months or years after their tour of duty is over. We discuss PTSD further in chapter 14.

It is not unusual for people to become anxious simply because they have had a brain injury and now must adjust to a new way of life. Symptoms of anxiety can also be due to side effects of medications, other medical conditions (thyroid problems, for example), substance abuse, or withdrawal from drugs such as alcohol, cocaine, or heroin. So, if anxiety persists, consult a physician for a thorough evaluation; don't just assume it is attributable to adjustment difficulties after the brain injury.

Treatment

As with other problems related to traumatic brain injury, a number of therapies are used to treat brain injury–induced anxiety.

Medication

Treatment for anxiety after brain injury often requires medications. Selective serotonin reuptake inhibitors (SSRIs) or serotonin norepinephrine reuptake inhibitors (SNRIs) are commonly used. SSRIs include Lexapro (escitalopram), Celexa (citalopram), and Zoloft (sertraline). Effexor (venlafaxine) is a commonly used SNRI. These drugs work well for long-term control of anxiety, but they can take a few weeks to work optimally. The benefit is that they have few major side effects and are not addictive. If SSRIs or SNRIs are ineffective, continue to work with your doctor, because there are other medications that can be used. However, in our opinion, it's best to avoid long-term use of benzodiazepines such as Valium (diazepam), Klonopin (clonazepam), or Ativan (lorazepam) because they can lead to addiction, cause memory problems, and interfere with gait and balance—and may paradoxically increase anxiety or agitation in some people.

Psychotherapy

Structured psychotherapeutic intervention is an effective treatment for anxiety, either by itself or in conjunction with medications. To participate in therapy, however, the person with brain injury must be able to understand and apply the training, a condition that makes talk therapy a better choice for those with mild to moderate brain injury. Certain forms of psychotherapy can be challenging for persons with severe brain injury, but with appropriate adjustments by the therapists, it can still be valuable.

Cognitive Behavioral Therapy

Cognitive behavioral therapy (CBT) focuses on understanding the links between feelings and behavior (as discussed in chapter 11). Typically, the person works with a therapist with expertise in cognitive behavioral therapy in regular weekly sessions for a few months. During these sessions, the therapist helps the person understand that their maladaptive behavior stems from beliefs that are counterproductive. The therapist typically assigns homework and asks the person to practice techniques outside the session. The overarching goal is not to focus on the past or on situations over which the person has no control, but instead to target the negative thought patterns and alter behavior. CBT teaches people to assess the validity of their thoughts and to replace unhelpful thoughts with more helpful ones. Thoughts, behaviors, and emotions are interrelated, but the feedback loop can be broken. An individual with anxiety appraises the world in a certain way, and adjustments to one's appraisal can change the anxious response. For example, an anxious person might feel slighted if someone they know walks by without acknowledging them. CBT would teach them to pause and consider other alternatives: perhaps the acquaintance literally may not have seen them or was lost in their own thoughts. CBT also teaches anxiety-reducing behavioral techniques such as deep breathing, meditation, creative visualization, and yoga.

Dialectical Behavioral Therapy and Other Therapies

Dialectical behavioral therapy (DBT, discussed in chapter 11) can also be an effective therapy for management of anxiety. PTSD-focused therapies include prolonged exposure (PE), cognitive processing therapy (CPT), and trauma-focused cognitive behavioral therapy (CBT). Ask your mental health professional about the best type of therapy for you.

Other Strategies

Other do-it-yourself strategies to cope with anxiety include maintaining a thought log and challenging dysfunctional/unhelpful thoughts and beliefs; maintaining a gratitude journal (writing every day at least one thing you are grateful for); regular physical exercise; and tai chi, qigong, or repetitive prayer. Cognitive exercises such as working on puzzles, playing board games, and working on arts and crafts can help alleviate anxiety.

Common problems following brain injury like memory deficits and poor organization skills can make anxiety worse. In these cases, learning strategies for supporting memory and other cognitive impairments can be very empowering and reduce anxiety.

In summary, anxiety after brain injury can be a significant problem. Some anxiety is healthy, but excessive anxiety can make life miserable and interfere with recovery from brain injury. The good news is that there are many treatment options for anxiety. A variety of medications is available to treat anxiety, and talk therapy and lifestyle strategies such as meditation and yoga are often helpful too. A combination of all these techniques may be the best route to resilience and optimal recovery from anxiety after brain injury.

Tips and tools on how to manage the symptoms discussed in this chapter appear in tables 13.1 and 13.2.

TABLE 13.1. TIPS AND TOOLS FOR COPING WITH ANXIETY AFTER BRAIN INJURY

Educate Yourself	Educate yourself about anxiety symptoms after brain injury.
	Learn to recognize your triggers.
Consult If Necessary	Consult a mental health professional if anxiety symptoms are persistent or distressing.
	Contact a psychiatrist, clinical psychologist, or a psychotherapist for help; any one of these clinicians can refer you to another clinician if you need more help than they can provide.
Accept the Situation	Accept your feelings and learn to manage them—having an anxiety disorder is not a sign of weakness or an embarrassment.
	You may feel that these symptoms will never go away, but know that anxiety is a treatable condition.
Follow Rules	Follow your clinicians' recommendations.
	Do not start, stop, or adjust medications without consulting your doctor.
	Stay away from alcohol and illicit drugs.
Practice	Practice makes perfect.
	Practice the anxiety-coping strategies your clinician recommends.

TABLE 13.2. TIPS AND TOOLS FOR CARING FOR SOMEONE EXPERIENCING ANXIETY AFTER BRAIN INJURY

It's Not about You	Do not take it personally.
	As a family member or caregiver, you may encounter some resistance to your well-meaning help and advice.
	Try not to be upset by the persistent anxiety, and do not take it personally when they get irritable or edgy.
Watch for Triggers	Be aware of topics/situations that trigger anxiety and try to avoid them.
	If the person talks about a trigger, listen to them.
Be a Pal	Practice calming activities such as deep breathing, meditation, or yoga with the person.
	Telling them to "get over it" is not helpful; it may be hard for them to disclose their fears if they feel you are judging them.
Be Available	Make yourself available.
	Not knowing where to go for help or whom to contact can worsen their anxiety.
	Letting the person with anxiety know that you are only a phone call away can be reassuring.
Take Care of Yourself	Get professional help if you yourself feel over-whelmed, anxious, or irritable in your role as caregiver.
	It is not uncommon for caregivers to be stressed by their caretaking duties, and it's crucial that you help yourself.

Take-Home Points

Anxiety is common after brain injury and can often occur independently or along with depression.

Symptoms can range from generalized free-floating anxiety to intense episodes that occur spontaneously or are triggered by real or perceived stress.

Treatment includes one or more of these: mind-body strategies (such as deep breathing, muscle relaxation, meditation, yoga), talk therapy, and/or medications.

Exercise

Whether you are a person with brain injury or a caregiver, you can try these simple exercises. There are also many apps and videos available. You can discuss with your mental health professional what would be the best for you.

Deep Breathing: The 4-4-6 Technique

• Sit or lie in a comfortable place.

• Put your hand on your belly and take a deep breath through your nose, counting to 4.

• Feel your hand on your belly rise.

• Hold your breath for about 4 seconds.

• Breathe out through your mouth counting to 6.

• Repeat for five to ten minutes until you feel calm.

Progressive Muscle Relaxation

• *Sit or lie in a comfortable place.*

• *Tense the muscles in your feet and inhale slowly (as above) through your nose.*

• *Hold your breath and keep the muscles of your feet tense for a few seconds.*

• *Slowly exhale through your mouth (as above) and release the muscle tension in your feet.*

• *Continue this exercise by working upward and focusing on one muscle group at a time.*

Guided Imagery

• *Sit or lie in a comfortable place.*

• *Start by taking a few deep breaths (as described above).*

• *Close your eyes and imagine a beautiful calming scene.*

• *Feel free to add appealing things to make it more calming and beautiful.*

• *Notice that you will slowly begin to relax and get less tense as you continue to imagine the beautiful scene.*

Chapter 14

PTSD

William, 34 years old, was involved in a three-car accident about four months ago. He lost consciousness for a few minutes after the accident. He was taken to a local hospital soon after the accident and had a medical workup and tests, all of which were normal, including computerized tomography (CT) of the head. He continued to have headaches, dizziness, and light and noise sensitivity, as well as visual problems for a few weeks after the accident. However, by the end of the month, he felt like himself again, except that he could not get the memory of the accident out of his mind. He started to have nightmares and flashbacks. Over the next few weeks, he even started to have intense memories of the accident to the point where he felt he could not drive. He stopped driving soon after, and his wife had to drive him around everywhere, including to his workplace.

PTSD (post-traumatic stress disorder) can occur after a brain injury of any severity. Unlike the other neuropsychiatric symptoms with brain injury that we have discussed so far, PTSD may not always be directly related to the physical impact of the brain injury. That is, it may not be due to the brain injury itself, but rather, it might be a possible outcome following a stressful event, such as a brain injury. However, brain injury can cause damage or dysfunction of certain brain regions such as the amygdala, hippocampus, and prefrontal cortex that can trigger symptoms of PTSD, or the injury can make the brain more vulnerable to react to stress.

PTSD is a set of symptoms that a person may experience after being exposed to, witnessing, or hearing about a traumatic event (such as death, sexual abuse, or physical violence), often with a sense of helplessness. It can manifest as four main sets of symptoms: intrusions, avoidance, negative emotions/thoughts, and hyperarousal. Intrusions refers to involuntarily reexperiencing a traumatic event (such as an accident, a fall, or combat). It could entail nightmares about what happened or even flashbacks, where the memory intrudes while awake, sometimes to the point where the person with the injury feels like they are reliving the incident. Avoidance refers to avoiding internal (memories, thoughts, feelings) and/or external (people, places, events) reminders of the traumatic event. Negative emotions/thoughts can include chronic sadness, lack of joy, and negative beliefs and distorted thinking of themselves, the world, or the future. Hyperarousal refers to an increase in the fight-or-flight system (arousal of the sympathetic nervous system) and can manifest as physical reactions such as increased heart rate or startle or insomnia, and in mood symptoms such as increased anxiety and irritability. A diagnosis of PTSD is made when symptoms last longer than one month. In general, they occur within three months of the traumatic event, but symptoms can occur much later.

PTSD can be debilitating after repeated reexperiencing of symptoms, negative emotionality, a frequent state of fight-or-flight, and consciously or subconsciously avoiding of memories, people, and places. PTSD is almost the opposite of dementia (where there is loss of memory); with PTSD, a traumatic memory is not forgettable but is potentially amplified in intensity. The memory is not just easily recollectable but also emotionally laden. PTSD can also occur in people who have no memory of the traumatic event. The amygdala is important in emotional memory and can be overactive in PTSD. Therefore, the memory creates a strong emotional reaction. There also can be decreased activity in the hippocampus (which stores and consolidates new learning and buffers the stress response) and in the ventromedial prefrontal cortex, which helps in eliminating the excess emotionality of memories. With PTSD, however, the ventromedial prefrontal cortex may not work optimally.

PTSD symptoms can overlap with other symptoms following the brain injury. With mild brain injury (such as William's at the beginning of the chapter), irritability and anxiety can occur due to the brain injury during the initial stages of recovery, but also can be due to PTSD later on. While these symptoms usually resolve over a few weeks or months, if they are due to PTSD, they may continue. It is thus important to recognize whether PTSD is part of the picture after brain injury.

Management

Once recognized, PTSD is treatable with therapy and medications, alone or in combination. The best treatment available today is a behavioral therapy called prolonged exposure (PE) therapy, whereby the person with PTSD is slowly and systematically exposed to the traumatic event. While this may sound cruel, it is based on the principle that the brain needs to learn that thinking about or being reminded about the traumatic event is not intolerable. In effect, the idea is to get the brain used to bringing up and dealing with the memory to the point where it is not such a big issue. Exposure therapy helps the brain's "alarm system" (including the amygdala and the hypothalamus and sympathetic nervous system) get attenuated with repeated exposures to the traumatic event.

Exposure therapy involves a therapist first collecting details about the traumatic event. The therapist then will get a sense on a Subjective Units of Distress (SUD) scale how distressing the memory is, often on a scale of 1 to 10, where 1 is minimal and 10 is maximal distress. Over time, the therapist will introduce elements of the memory and keep exposing these elements until the SUD is lowered. After this exposure, the therapist may introduce another element of the memory and keep doing this until the SUD for this added memory is lowered.

In William's case from the beginning of the chapter, for example, the therapist may start with a picture of cars on the road. This may be overwhelming to William, with a SUD of 10. Over repeated sessions, the therapist could show this picture and discuss it until William rates the SUD as much lower. At this point, William has become tolerant to the picture of cars on the road. As a next step, the therapist may show William a video of someone driving on an icy road and having a fender bender. Again, William may find this overwhelming at first, but over time, he will be able to tolerate it. As a final step, the therapist may actually have William drive a car. Again, this may have to be done repetitively until William becomes tolerant to it. Exposure therapy targets one of the main problems with PTSD, the natural inclination to avoid thinking about or remembering the trauma. Unfortunately, avoidance can lead to perpetuating the PTSD symptoms.

There are many other therapies for PTSD, such as cognitive processing therapy (CPT) and eye movement desensitization and reprocessing (EMDR).

CPT is a specific type of cognitive behavioral therapy where the person learns how to identify and challenge unhealthy and negative beliefs associated with traumatic experience and create a new narrative of the experience that can be more helpful and healthy. EMDR is a form of trauma therapy where eye movements are used to process the traumatic experience and in so doing reduce the distress associated with the experience.

It is important that the person discuss with their therapist the best treatment option given the symptoms and distress.

Medication

Another treatment for PTSD is medications, particularly selective serotonin reuptake inhibitors (SSRIs). Sertraline and paroxetine are two such medications that are approved by the FDA for PTSD treatment. These medications can help with the excessive emotional reaction to the trauma by reducing activity in the brain's "alarm system" (particularly the amygdala). The goal of medication (and exposure therapy) is to reduce the excessive anxiety due to the traumatic memory, not to get rid of the memory itself. With successful treatment, the memory will still be there, but it will cease to have such a powerful hold on the person.

Prazosin is a medication that is often prescribed to treat nightmares associated with PTSD. Even though some studies have found it to be effective, others have not. Talk to your doctor about which medications are most likely to help you.

In summary, PTSD can pose a roadblock to full recovery. It can confuse the clinical picture after a brain injury, because some of the symptoms can overlap. Furthermore, untreated PTSD can even prolong the effects of symptoms that were initially associated with the brain injury. It is important to recognize PTSD, especially since it is treatable with therapy and medications.

Tips and tools on how to manage the symptoms discussed in this chapter appear in tables 14.1 and 14.2.

TABLE 14.1. TIPS AND TOOLS FOR COPING WITH PTSD AFTER BRAIN INJURY	
Educate Yourself	Find a professional who is knowledgeable about brain injury and PTSD and learn about your symptoms and their impact on your life.
Practice Self-Soothing Strategies	In addition to practicing strategies you've learned from your therapist, you can also try simple self-soothing strategies to cope with your anxiety such as taking a warm bath, listening to music, sipping a hot cup of herbal tea, taking a walk, and just breathing fresh air—strategies that may distract your brain from focusing on the trauma.
Learn about Your Triggers	Make a note of all your triggers.
	Talk to people who care for you about your triggers so that they can support you and help you limit your exposure to them.
	Your clinician will also teach you other ways to cope with your triggers.

Table 14.1 continued on next page

Practice Healthy Living	Stay away from alcohol and illicit drugs, as they can make your symptoms worse.
	Exercise regularly.
	Practice sleep hygiene.
	Eat healthy meals.
	Contact your doctor if you have any other medical issues.
	Find hobbies and other healthy social distractions.
Find a Support Group	Participating in a support group gives you an opportunity to talk about your symptoms if you choose and to learn from others who have also experienced some type of brain trauma on how they are coping with symptoms; it also helps you realize that you are not alone and that help is available.

TABLE 14.2. TIPS AND TOOLS FOR CARING FOR SOMEONE WITH PTSD AFTER BRAIN INJURY

Get Professional Help	Encourage the person to obtain professional help; people with PTSD may be embarrassed about their symptoms or feel guilty and not seek professional help.
	PTSD is a treatable condition, and help is available.
Be Available	People with PTSD often feel alone. Because of their feelings of guilt, embarrassment, and shame, they often withdraw and isolate themselves.
	Knowing that they have someone they can trust and someone who does not judge them and is supportive can be invaluable for them.
Understand Their Triggers	Talk to the person about their triggers.
	Once the triggers are identified, make a plan with the person for how to limit their exposure to the triggers, and practice strategies with them that they learned in therapy.
	Do NOT do exposure therapy with them.

Listen; Don't Judge	Allow the person to talk about their trauma at a pace they are a comfortable with. Don't push or pressure. Let them take their time.
	Negative emotions such as anger and irritability may surface. Allow them to express them, but ensure safety.
	Do not judge them, blame them, or minimize their traumatic experience.

Take-Home Points

PTSD can occur after a traumatic event, such as a brain injury of any severity.

PTSD can involve four main sets of symptoms: intrusions, avoidance, negative emotions, and hyperarousal.

PTSD is a treatable condition and often requires a combination of medications and therapy.

Initially experiencing an emotional reaction after a trauma is normal; however, when it persists past a month and affects one's daily life, PTSD should be a diagnostic consideration.

Exercise

Do it yourself: use PTSD as an acronym to cope with trauma and its associated problems.

Practice a healthy lifestyle.

Therapy: Seek professional help from therapists with expertise in management of trauma.

Support: Join a PTSD support group and increase socialization.

Develop: Develop healthy ways to calm and distract yourself such as exercise, hobbies, or outdoor activities.

Part IV

Behavioral Disorders Caused *by the* Traumatized Brain

In this part of the book, we explore behavioral changes that often occur after brain injury. These behavioral issues can include psychosis (chapter 15), aggression (chapter 16), impulsivity (chapter 17), substance use disorders (chapter 18), apathy (lack of motivation) (chapter 19), and sleep disturbances (chapter 20). Behavioral issues can be a serious concern for family members of a person who has had brain injury. Not only can the behavioral issues cause problems within the family, but they may affect recovery from the brain injury. While physical injuries are obvious, behavioral issues may be hidden in some ways. Behavioral changes after brain injury may be unexpected, or there may be a failure to recognize or make the connection between the behavior and the brain injury. Such misunderstandings can make behavioral changes after brain injury especially troubling.

Chapter 15

Psychosis

isa worked hard and saved for her dream vacation—a ski trip to the Colorado Rockies with three close friends to celebrate her twenty-seventh birthday. On their last day on the slopes, Lisa collided with another skier and slammed the side of her head into a tree. She was airlifted to the emergency department of a nearby hospital and diagnosed with severe traumatic brain injury. Once she was stable, Lisa was transported to her hometown hospital, where she participated in several weeks of rehabilitation. Not long after she returned home to her parents and younger brother, she developed seizures, for which her doctor prescribed an anti-seizure medication.

About a year after the accident, Lisa began having suspicious thoughts that an old high school teacher was going to kill her and her family. She became convinced that she had to perform several rituals to keep the teacher away from her loved ones. Among the actions she felt compelled to do were to spit in the sink in a certain pattern when brushing her teeth, place eggshells on the kitchen counter in a line, and arrange magazines in a certain way on the dining room table. Her family was puzzled at first and then grew frustrated by her compulsion to perform these rituals. Her mother explained to Lisa's doctor that Lisa had had no contact or communication with the teacher for many years.

An injury to the brain can trigger the onset of psychosis sometimes even in an individual with no history of prior psychosis. The words *psycho-*

sis and *psychotic symptoms* refer to delusions, hallucinations, or illogical thinking. In other words, psychosis is a state in which the sufferer is not in touch with what others would agree is reality. In this chapter, we discuss the various forms psychotic symptoms can take after brain injury.

Symptoms

Delusions are fixed false beliefs that a person firmly holds, despite evidence to the contrary. For example, Lisa in our opening story had delusions that her old teacher was going to kill her and her family. Lisa firmly believed this, even though she had not heard from the teacher for years and despite repeated assurances from her family that there was no threat. She also held the firm belief that, by arranging things in certain ways, she could prevent the teacher from harming her or her family.

Paranoid delusions, in particular, are typical of psychosis after brain injury. Just as in Lisa's case, people with paranoid delusions have the unshakable belief that someone is watching them or targeting them, even if there is no evidence to support that belief. People who have paranoid delusions are convinced that their lives are in danger, that they must always be vigilant, and that they are at risk of significant bodily harm. Cognitive deficits can add to such paranoia. For example, if a person with paranoia can't remember where they placed certain things (keys or a purse, for instance), their paranoia can escalate into believing that someone is entering their house and stealing those items from them.

Psychosis can also include hallucinations. A person who hallucinates sees, hears, smells, or feels things that are not in our consensual reality, but those hallucinations are as real to them as anything else in their experience. As we discussed in chapter 6, the brain takes in sensory information and constructs a model of reality. If there is brain injury, the brain's model of reality can change, leading to perceptions others do not experience. These perceptions can be frightening and can lead to agitation and anxiety. The most common type of hallucinations after

brain injury are auditory hallucinations, often consisting of conversations between two people about them. Such hallucinations may consist
of hearing people arguing about them or mumbling in a way that they
cannot fully understand. If they overhear an imagined "conversation"
coming from another room, they may go to investigate and discover no
one there. They may hear inanimate objects such as a lamp, a desk, or
even the carpet speaking to them.

Illogical thinking, in which thoughts are jumbled or disorganized, is
another form of psychosis. The person with brain injury who experiences this jumbled thinking usually does not complain about the symptoms
for the simple reason that they are not aware that there's a problem.
Family members usually take the person to a doctor when they notice
the strange behavior. The illogical thinking may be so severe that others
cannot understand what the person is saying.

Other symptoms of psychosis include odd behavior such as hold-
ing a two-way conversation with oneself, laughing, or grinning inappropriately, or a sudden behavioral change—withdrawing socially or
ignoring personal hygiene, for example. Confabulation is a symptom
that sometimes can be mistaken for psychosis. People who confabulate
often make up stories to fill in gaps in their memory. Confabulation can
appear as delusion, but it is a different phenomenon stemming from
profound memory problems.

Risk Factors

Psychotic symptoms are more common in people who have had brain
injuries, particularly those with severe TBIs, compared with those who
have not. Psychosis may be more likely after TBI if the brain was vulnerable because of preexisting brain damage associated with birth or a
learning disability, even if relatively mild. Other factors that increase
the risk of psychosis after traumatic brain injury are traumatic brain
injury in early childhood and a personal or family history of psychosis
or schizophrenia.

Some people who develop psychotic symptoms after brain injury have a family history of a psychotic disorder like schizophrenia or had milder psychotic symptoms before the brain injury. Similarly, having a brain injury elevates the risk for developing schizophrenia in those who have a family history of schizophrenia, particularly if that person is a first-degree relative (parent, child, or sibling) of the person with schizophrenia.

The strongest of these risk factors is the severity of the brain injury; people with severe brain injury are far more likely to have psychosis than those with mild brain injury. And the more severe the brain injury, the greater the likelihood of having seizures—and having seizures further increases the risk of psychotic symptoms.

Some people with psychosis after brain injury may not develop the full spectrum of schizophrenia symptoms (including hallucinations and delusions) but develop only what are called negative symptoms, including lack of motivation, poor thinking skills, lack of speech, and lack of emotion. Other people with brain injury do not develop these negative symptoms but experience only delusions, such as believing that family members are not who they are, but are impostors (Capgras syndrome), or beliefs such as that a particular location has been duplicated and is present in two different sites (reduplicative paramnesia).

The timing of post–brain injury psychosis varies. Sometimes psychosis develops immediately after the brain injury and often in the context of delirium. People experiencing delirium become confused as to where they are and what is happening to them. They may have frightening visual hallucinations: they may see armies marching into their hospital room threatening to shoot them or fantastical animals flying in the room, perhaps chimeras, who transform themselves into monsters with gnashing teeth. They may see hospital staff stealthily mixing poison into their intravenous fluids. They may see their caregivers transforming into demons, ready to eviscerate them. Such hallucinations can be terrifying, even overwhelming, for the person with brain injury.

Psychotic symptoms in the context of delirium can stem from multiple factors. In some cases, the brain injury itself is the direct cause.

Alternatively, certain medications, lack of oxygen, and several concurrent medical problems like blood loss or anemia can also cause delirium. Scientists believe that delirium develops in response to a decrease in a brain chemical called acetylcholine. This chemical is also important for dreaming. If we consider delirium as a dream state, in which dreams mix with consciousness, it may be a state of consciousness between wakefulness and dreaming. Delirium tends to wax and wane, and in most cases when the cause is identified and treated appropriately, delirium will resolve.

Psychotic symptoms can also develop months or years after a brain injury. It is not clear why this happens, although it seems that people who have injuries to the temporal lobe may be more prone to this later onset. It may be that as the brain reorganizes after the injury, faulty "rewiring" allows psychotic symptoms to occur. There is evidence, in fact, that dysfunction of the white matter (the axon tracts that connect different parts of the brain) is related to psychotic symptoms. Injury to these tracts could lead to poor crosstalk between sections of the brain and eventually to psychosis.

Damage to the frontal lobes, basal ganglia, and hippocampi is also associated with psychosis (see figures 2.1a and b). The hippocampi, seahorse-shaped structures deep within the brain inside the temporal lobes, are important in retaining short-term memory. It is also clear, however, that the hippocampi are smaller than normal in people who have schizophrenia, and damage to the hippocampus may be related to psychosis.

Lisa in our opening story had severe brain injury, seizures, and psychosis in the form of persecution-type delusions that developed several months after her injury. Her case is a typical presentation of psychosis after brain injury.

Management

People with brain injury who experience hallucinations or delusions should undergo a thorough medical evaluation, including a magnetic resonance imaging (MRI) of the brain and an electroencephalogram (EEG), a recording of the electrical activity in the brain. The doctor will note what medications the patient is taking, to rule out either medications or concurrent medical problems as the source of the delirium. The doctor will also take steps to rule out substance use disorder, because certain drugs of abuse can cause or worsen psychotic symptoms. Cocaine, amphetamines, methamphetamines, LSD, Ecstasy, "bath salts," and marijuana, among others, can cause psychotic symptoms. In addition, the doctor will also ask questions about the person's birth, early childhood, social and environmental conditions, and any family history of psychosis.

If the person with brain injury exhibits psychotic symptoms, they are not being purposefully difficult. The person is likely agitated because their hallucinations are frightening to them. They may believe that their caregiver or family is trying to harm them and so may lash out or resist help.

Antipsychotic medications are commonly prescribed to treat psychosis. Examples include Risperdal (risperidone), Haldol (haloperidol), Zyprexa (olanzapine), Seroquel (quetiapine), Abilify (aripiprazole), Latuda (lurasidone), and Clozaril (clozapine). There is some evidence in the literature to suggest that haloperidol interferes with neuronal recovery in people with brain injury and therefore is best avoided. Antipsychotic medications work by lowering the amount of a neurotransmitter in the brain called dopamine. A simplistic explanation is that excess dopamine in one particular tract of the brain is associated with the production of psychotic symptoms.

Unfortunately, persons with psychotic symptoms often have poor insight into their condition. In other words, they may not think there is anything wrong with them, or they may believe that they can deal with the situation on their own. In either case, they may not want to take their medication. If you are a caregiver, emphasize to the person you are caring for just how important it is that they take the antipsychotic medication, at least for the short term. People with brain injury may have psychotic symptoms for the short term and may not have to be on antipsychotic medications permanently.

Arguing with a person who is experiencing psychosis about their beliefs is unproductive and can even lead to agitation. Delusions are by definition fixed, and it is unlikely that you will be successful in convincing the person that their beliefs are false. The same is true for hallucinations; after all, to the person who sees or hears them, the hallucinations are real.

As family, friend, or caregiver, you can best serve the person by being understanding and supportive and by encouraging them to take their medications and to follow their doctor's advice. You do not have to agree with their beliefs but you can validate their distress and help them cope with their anxiety.

It can be disheartening to see your family member in the hospital because of psychosis. They may beg and plead for you to get them out. Understand that they are in the hospital for good reasons. Today, most hospital stays are short, a few days to a week or two.

In summary, psychosis after brain injury can occur, but it is less likely to develop than depression or anxiety. Psychotic symptoms may develop after the injury as part of an acute confusional state or they may develop months to years later. Luckily, medications are available to reduce these symptoms quite effectively. Dealing with someone who has psychotic symptoms can be distressing, but it may be reassuring to hear that many people do get better with the appropriate treatment. Understanding that psychosis is in some way connected to their brain injury can help you, as a caregiver, empathize and be supportive to the person you are caring for.

Tips and tools on how to manage the symptoms discussed in this chapter appear in tables 15.1 and 15.2.

TABLE 15.1. TIPS AND TOOLS FOR COPING WITH PSYCHOSIS AFTER BRAIN INJURY

Comply with Medical Advice	Take your medications as prescribed and follow recommendations of the health professionals taking care of you.
Seek Comfort	Do not isolate yourself.
	Stay in touch with people who comfort you.
	Maintain contact with family and friends, people you can talk to when stressed and who can reassure you.
Check with Loved Ones	Don't always go by your feelings. Check with your loved one if you believe you may be overthinking. Have a go-to person or group that you can connect with when feeling out of sorts.
Have a Support Kit	Create a support kit—a list of usually pleasurable activities you can do to distract yourself when you get anxious or have distressing thoughts.
	You can connect with your go-to person and distract yourself with one of your pleasurable activities. This usually helps.

TABLE 15.2. TIPS AND TOOLS FOR CARING FOR SOMEONE WITH PSYCHOSIS AFTER BRAIN INJURY

Educate Yourself	Educate yourself about psychosis.
	Learn about the symptoms, medications, triggers for relapse, and people or physicians to call in case of an emergency.
Emphasize Safety	If you are concerned about the safety of the person, take them to the nearest hospital or call 911.
	When calling 911, ask for the mobile crisis team or the officer on duty for the crisis intervention team, if available.

Respond to Their Feelings, Not Their Beliefs	If the person is describing abnormal experiences, respond to their feelings, not their words. They may be frightened.
	You may feel you are tricking the person or lying to them by not correcting their thinking. It is more productive to reframe their thinking and focus on supporting their emotions.
Keep Your Goal Simple	Your goal is to provide comfort and support.
	The goal is not to make the person understand the truth, for psychosis eliminates their ability to appreciate the truth.
	The goal is to make the person feel safe and less distressed.
	Redirecting their focus to relaxing activities can distract them from their tormenting thoughts.
Don't Argue	Never argue with a person with brain injury psychosis. Trying to convince them that it is all in their mind or calling them crazy is counterproductive and may only make them more agitated and even aggressive.

Take-Home Points

Psychotic symptoms can happen after brain injury.

Psychosis can present in many forms: delusions, hallucinations, disorganized thinking, negative symptoms.

Psychosis can be time limited (such as during an episode of delirium) or more persistent.

Psychosis can emerge at different points in recovery.

Psychosis is a treatable condition. If you are concerned about safety of the person or others, call 911.

Exercise

Do not despair if your symptoms are not under control. Continue to talk to your doctor about other medications and alternative treatments.

*Meanwhile, keep up with **S-E-L-F C-A-R-E**:*

S *Sleep hygiene*

E *Exercise regularly*

L *Learn something that's new or appealing to you*

F *Fun and enjoyable activities participation*

C *Connect with family, friends, loved ones*

A *Avoid recreational drugs*

R *Routinize your days*

E *Eat healthy*

Chapter 16

Aggression

Lee was in his early 60s and was diagnosed with high blood pressure about 15 years ago. He was advised by his doctor to take medication and also make some changes to his lifestyle—including exercising regularly, reducing his weight (he was more than 15 pounds above his expected body weight), eating healthily, and stopping smoking. He tried to make some changes but struggled to maintain a healthier lifestyle. One day, he woke up with a severe headache, which he described as the worst headache of his life. He vomited a few times and seemed very drowsy and lethargic. His wife immediately called 911, and the paramedics rushed him to the hospital. Medical workup revealed that he had a ruptured aneurysm (an aneurysm is a ballooning of a blood vessel in the brain), which had caused bleeding in the brain and a subarachnoid hemorrhage (bleeding in the space surrounding the brain). The doctors recommended immediate surgery. The surgery was successful, but it was followed by a prolonged hospital stay, followed by extensive rehabilitation. While in the hospital, Lee developed seizures and had episodes of agitation immediately after he was admitted, but both conditions resolved over time.

After Lee returned home, he had emotional outbursts over trivial matters. For example, a minor disagreement at the dinner table with his family escalated into a shouting match, and Lee stormed off, punching holes in walls. At one point, Lee became so enraged over an empty cereal box that he wrenched the cupboard door off its hinges. Lee's wife reported, "The grandchildren are terrified of him now." Because of these aggressive episodes, it has been hard for Lee to get into a day program whose goal is to help him transition back to work.

Symptoms

Aggression is hostile, harmful, or destructive behavior that can be physical or verbal and can range from irritability to physical assault on others. Aggression can manifest as cursing, threatening, hitting, pushing, yelling, or breaking or throwing things. Physical aggression, in particular, can be disturbing to caregivers and disruptive to recovery for the person with brain injury. An outburst of aggression from a previously calm person may be scary for caregivers to deal with. Aggression may also frighten the person with brain injury; they may feel out of control and scared. People who develop aggression after brain injury may need to be medicated, perhaps even placed in a medical facility for monitoring. For you, as a caregiver or support person, to provide the best support for the person with aggression, you must understand how aggression can occur after brain injury and how best to manage it, for your own safety and the safety of others.

Aggression is a possible outcome after brain injury. It is more common after repeated brain injuries and after severe injuries. Risk factors for developing aggression include being male, repeated brain injuries, severe brain injury, injury to the frontal lobes, use of alcohol or illicit drugs, and the onset of mood problems after the injury. Alcohol or illicit drug use after brain injury can release inhibitions, making the person with brain injury more vulnerable to acting out aggressively.

Certain patterns and features tend to occur with aggressive behavior after brain injury. The aggression typically is reactive, that is, triggered by a specific thing or event, even a very minor stressor. In Lee's case, in our opening story, trivial disagreements made him agitated and aggressive. The aggressive reaction can be entirely disproportionate to the issue at hand.

Aggressive behaviors after brain injury tend to be impulsive. Typically, the person with brain injury doesn't mull over a perceived slight, start getting angry, and then plan what to say or do. Rather, the response to a trigger is sudden and explosive, without gradual buildup. Aggression after brain injury is thus not criminal violence, in which criminals plot and plan, execute a crime, then make their planned escape. However, it is important to remember that brain injury explains the aggressive behavior but does not excuse it; this is why appropriate treatment is so important.

Just as aggression after brain injury typically erupts suddenly, it also dies down abruptly; it is not usually sustained. Indeed, people with brain injury usually regret their outburst. They tend to be embarrassed and upset by their own behavior. They tend not to blame others and do not justify their behavior.

Aggression can occur soon after brain injury or months later. Aggression soon after the brain injury, in the context of confusion and disorientation, is most likely due to delirium (an acute confusional state triggered by any number of causes such as medications or surgery). This aggressive behavior is the direct result of the trauma to the brain and the subsequent alterations in body physiology or of medications administered after the brain injury, such as pain medications. In the context of delirium, the person's thinking is muddled; the person may be confused about where they are or what happened. This uncertainty may fluctuate; they may seem "with it" at times and completely confused at other times. When they are confused, they may act out aggressively to defend themselves. They may believe they are in the middle of a war zone or in a fantastical world of demons. They may have visual hallucinations, perhaps seeing frightening displays of aggression by imagined monsters.

In a hospital setting, aggression due to delirium is usually treated with medication. Doctors use these medications temporarily while the brain recovers from the immediate shock of the trauma. The brain injury can also cause other medical problems, which can also cause delirium. Infections can develop, sodium or calcium or magnesium levels can be abnormal, or blood oxygen levels can fall. Treating and resolving these issues can help manage the delirium, but doctors often use antipsychotic

medications as well. If required, antipsychotics are necessary for a limited time, as they can be necessary to reduce the aggression and make sure
no one (including the person with brain injury) is harmed. They may
also potentially reduce the duration of the delirium, though this theory
is controversial.

Medications can also lead to delirium, and the doctor will evaluate
any medications the person with brain injury is taking. Certain medicines that reduce a neurotransmitter called acetylcholine are particularly
important to investigate because they can cause delirium. These include
medicines like Benadryl (diphenhydramine) or bladder medications
like Ditropan (oxybutynin), among many others. If the person with
brain injury was drinking large quantities of alcohol before the injury,
they may be in alcohol withdrawal, which can certainly cause aggression. People who were regularly taking benzodiazepines, such as Ativan
(lorazepam), Xanax (alprazolam), or Klonopin (clonazepam), before the
injury may also experience withdrawal. A person going through withdrawal from alcohol or benzodiazepines may be restless, sweating, shaky,
and sensitive to light or sound, have a rapid heartbeat or high blood
pressure, or hallucinate. Withdrawal from pain medicines (opiates like
Vicodin, OxyContin, or Percocet) can also cause agitation and aggression. Drugs like cocaine, amphetamines, or phencyclidine (PCP) can
cause aggression as well.

After a brain injury, seizures can occur, and seizures may be associated with or followed by aggression. In general, if related to seizures,
the aggression is brief and not directed toward anyone. Other causes
of aggression soon after a brain injury include metabolic disturbances
such as low blood sugar or change in blood electrolytes, such as sodium
levels. The doctors will investigate all these possibilities as causes for
the aggression. Sometimes it is not just one thing but a combination of
things that leads to delirium and aggression.

After the acute brain injury period, the person may develop aggression for many other reasons. They might be susceptible to other medical problems; for example, they may be vulnerable to falls and sustain
another brain injury. They could develop significant depression and

manifest their internal psychic pain physically as aggression. They may develop severe anxiety and lash out at people or things because they have trouble expressing their anger. They may have nightmares or recurrent thoughts of the incident associated with brain injury and develop PTSD. Pain that follows a brain injury can also cause agitation and aggression. Trouble adjusting to a new level of functioning, becoming dependent on family or friends, or feeling sorry for themselves and bitter about what fate has dealt them—all these swirling emotions can lead to aggression in the person with brain injury. People with personality traits of increased impulsivity and low frustration tolerance are also likely to get aggressive and indulge in violent behaviors, which puts them at risk for sustaining more brain injuries, which in turn can exacerbate aggression. Finally, the brain injury itself can affect parts of the brain that control emotions, including anger, and lead to long-term problems with aggression.

Damage to specific areas of the brain leads to aggression (see figures 2.1a and b). The frontal lobes and temporal lobes are prone to injury after physical trauma to the head, and these are the very areas critical to controlling our impulses to anger. Damage to the lower part of the frontal lobes (the orbitofrontal part of the prefrontal cortex) and the front of the temporal lobes (the anterior temporal lobes) is most closely associated with aggression. The amygdala, within the emotional brain (or limbic system), is also important for aggression and is involved in emotional regulation. Activation of the amygdala can spark outrage or an exaggerated response to perceived slights—exactly the form of aggression often seen after brain injury. Finally, the hypothalamus may play a role in aggression because it is responsible for fight-or-flight reactions; stimulation of areas in the hypothalamus can also lead to aggressive behavior.

There might be a circuit involving the orbitofrontal cortex, anterior temporal lobe, amygdala, and hypothalamus that is critical in controlling our aggressive impulses (figure 16.1). The aggressive impulses generated by the amygdala and the hypothalamus are probably normally regulated by the orbitofrontal cortex and perhaps the anterior temporal lobe. In other words, these cortical areas of the brain may act as a kind of brake on the aggressive impulses of the emotional brain. Damage to these frontal or temporal areas deactivates the brake, as it were, setting loose the emotional brain's aggressive impulses.

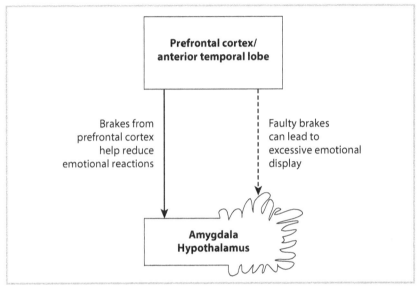

Figure 16.1. The Brain's Regulation of Emotions

On another level, we can look at the neurotransmitters that are associated with aggression. Norepinephrine, dopamine, serotonin, acetylcholine, and GABA may all play roles in aggressive behavior. Increased norepinephrine or dopamine, or decreased serotonin or GABA, can be associated with aggression. There might also be a genetic predisposition to aggression after brain injury expressed by a gene for an enzyme called monoamine oxidase type A (MAO-A). This enzyme is important in breaking down dopamine, norepinephrine, and serotonin. People who have a genetic predilection for low levels of MAO-A may be more likely to be aggressive when provoked, presumably because they cannot break down some of these neurotransmitters (particularly norepinephrine and dopamine) effectively.

Management

The best treatment for aggression depends on whether the aggression is acute or chronic. Acute aggression lasts up to a few weeks, whereas chronic aggression extends beyond that. Chronic aggression can be particularly challenging.

Environmental and Behavioral Therapies and Lifestyle Changes

In treating chronic aggression after brain injury, non-pharmacological approaches are an important part of treatment. Cognitive behavioral therapy (CBT) can help the person with brain injury improve their coping skills, making it easier for them to manage their frustration. CBT also helps with depression and anxiety, both of which may be contributing to aggression. Of course, the person with brain injury must have the cognitive abilities to benefit from CBT. CBT can also teach caregivers the coping skills they need to overcome their own frustrations as they try to help the person with aggression.

For people who have severe brain injury, behavioral and environmental interventions are critical. These approaches involve assessing the **a**ntecedents to the behavior, the **b**ehavior itself, and the **c**onsequences of the behavior, also known as the ABCs of assessing behavior problems. Assessing the antecedents involves careful history taking and observations. Does it seem that the person with brain injury is getting aggressive because they are not able to communicate properly? Do they get aggressive only with certain caregivers? If so, is it because those caregivers invade their personal space, for example? Could the physical environment or some discomfort be making them aggressive? Is their environment overstimulating them? Are they uncomfortable or in pain and have no way to express that other than aggression?

Assessing the aggressive behavior itself means observing the pattern in the behavior. Is the aggression verbal or physical? Does the person appear fearful? Could they be hallucinating? Or does the lashing out occur only when someone touches them? Is it when they have night-mares? Is it when they do not sleep well?

The final step is to explore the consequences of the behavior. Some-times caregivers may be inadvertently encouraging the aggression. For example, if the person with brain injury doesn't get much attention except when they are aggressive, getting that attention, even if it is neg-ative attention, may encourage the behavior further. If the aggression reflects hunger, pain, or a need to use the toilet, simply reassuring or redirecting the person may increase aggression because the underlying issue has not been addressed.

Therapists who specialize in working with people who have brain injury are most qualified to perform these behavioral and environmen-tal interventions, but caregivers/support persons should be aware of these principles as well. The professional may create a plan—in a reha-bilitation setting, for example—and it is up to caregivers to implement the plan when the person with brain injury returns home.

Medication

Aggression in the acute stage (which often stems from delirium) is treat-ed with medications determined by the treating doctor. Benzodiazepines such as Ativan (lorazepam) may be used because they work quickly and are calming. However, it's best to avoid benzodiazepines except where alcohol or benzodiazepine withdrawal is responsible for the aggression. Benzodiazepines can cause problems such as confusion, grogginess, or poor coordination and have the potential for addiction. In people with brain injury, benzodiazepines may also paradoxically worsen agitation.

There are medications for chronic aggression, and doctors often prescribe them in combination with the behavioral and environmen-tal techniques discussed above. Beta blockers (which treat high blood pressure and cardiac issues), particularly Inderal (propranolol), are the most effective drugs for chronic aggression. Be aware, however, that it often takes weeks for these medications to take effect, and the doctor may need to adjust the dose several times to find the correct level for your loved one.

Antidepressants like Zoloft (sertraline), Celexa (citalopram), and Lexapro (escitalopram) may be helpful, not only for those with depression or anxiety along with the aggression, but also for their general effects on aggression. Buspar (buspirone) an antianxiety agent, also seems to have anti-aggression effects in persons with brain injury.

Anticonvulsant medications can also be helpful, as they assist in stabilizing mood. Tegretol (carbamazepine) in particular seems to be beneficial. The doctor may also consider using Depakote (valproic acid). These medications help people with brain injury who may have seizures associated with the injury, but they can also help with aggression even when there are no seizures.

Stimulants like Ritalin (methylphenidate) can be used, with caution, in certain cases. However, they can also worsen aggression in some people. Finally, antipsychotic medications may be used in the long term for aggression as well, although they are best used when psychotic symptoms coincide with the aggression.

In summary, aggression after brain injury can be disconcerting to all involved. Family and caregivers must recognize that aggression after brain injury is often a consequence of factors beyond a person's control. As we have noted, there are multiple potential causes of the aggression, ranging from direct effects of the brain injury, other medical issues, medications, and illicit drugs to adjustment and social factors. A number of pharmacological and non-pharmacological options are available to help control this behavior. Managing the aggression will allow the person with brain injury to make a better recovery, stay at home, and return more quickly to a higher functioning level. With the help of physicians, therapists, and other specialists, you can help the person with brain injury and aggression overcome this behavior.

Tips and tools on how to manage the symptoms discussed in this chapter appear in tables 16.1 and 16.2.

TABLE 16.1. TIPS AND TOOLS FOR COPING WITH AGGRESSION AFTER BRAIN INJURY

Learn to Press the Pause Button	A good way of controlling your urges to speak or act is by learning to press the pause button.
	You are more likely to be heard, understood, and followed when you pause and think and express your concerns in a nonconfrontational way.
Find a Healthy Outlet	Find a healthy outlet to release your anger. It can be anything that comes easily to you that is safe and enjoyable. Examples include taking a walk, singing, listening to music, or finding something funny to say.
Get Help	If you are having difficulty controlling your emotions, get professional help.

TABLE 16.2. TIPS AND TOOLS FOR CARING FOR SOMEONE WITH AGGRESSION AFTER BRAIN INJURY

Emphasize Safety	Safety comes first, the safety of the person experiencing aggression and that of those around them.
	If the aggression escalates and the person cannot calm down, call 911 or get immediate help.
Respond but Don't React	Do your best to respond to the person with aggression calmly and gently, speaking softly but clearly, while ensuring that the environment is safe.
	Take pauses before speaking and focus on being nonreactive.
Watch for Triggers	Be alert for aggression triggers and try to minimize or remove them.
	Triggers may be related to the environment (such as too much noise, bright lights, cluttered space), people (loud conversations, too many directions given at once), or lifestyle (using alcohol or illicit drugs, sleeping poorly, taking certain medications).

	During calm moments, ask the patient what the triggers are; open up communication.
Teach	Identify behavioral patterns of aggression. Channel the aggressive energy into healthier, safer activity. For example, if the person with aggression likes to throw things when they get aggressive, give them a soft, squishy ball or a pillow and teach them to squeeze it when they feel angry.
	Teach them this behavior when they are calm and willing to listen and learn.
	During an aggressive outburst, people are usually unable to learn any new techniques.
Discuss Consequences	Discuss the consequences of aggressive behavior with the person with aggression.
	Pick a time when they are calm to discuss their behavior and state specific consequences of such behavior: "If you ever threaten the children, I'll ask you to leave the house."
	Be consistent with consequences, because inconsistent responses are confusing and can interfere with learning behavioral change.
Think outside the Box	Be creative; if the coping strategies you have devised just aren't working, keep searching for other methods to use.
	Seek guidance and help from doctors, therapists, or support groups.

Take-Home Points

Aggressive behaviors after brain injury tend to be impulsive, without planning or forethought, and reactive, reacting to real or perceived stress.

Aggression is usually intermittent and transient, and the person feels remorseful after the outburst.

Work out the ABCs of aggression (Antecedent, Behavior, Consequences)—consider mapping it out on paper.

A number of medication and non-medication options are available to help control aggression. You should consult with your health professional about them.

Exercise

*Aggression and anger can feel overwhelming. Sometimes it really helps to **STOP**.*

• **S**top; pause what you are doing. We all just need to slow down and stop sometimes. It may feel hard, but practice helps.

• **T**ake a deep breath. Close your eyes and take a deep breath through your nose into your belly counting to 4. Expand your belly like a balloon. Hold your breath for 4 seconds and then exhale slowly through your mouth allowing your belly to go inward, counting to 6. Take several breaths to calm your respiratory and heart rate. Allow your nervous system a moment to calm down.

• **O**bserve what is happening around and inside of you. Notice how tight your body feels and what your emotions are. Notice that the argument you are in is not getting you to the solution you had wanted. Think about what you are observing. Are you just not going to get to a point of agreement? Take time to really evaluate what is happening. Think about being responsive and not reactive.

• **P**roceed with the moment, the day, the situation. It may be that you pivot or change your behavior, or simply that you have allowed yourself a moment to be more thoughtful about your words.

Chapter 17

Impulsivity

Kayla is 54 and an avid tennis player. While reaching to return a serve one morning, she stumbled, tripped, and fell sideways on the edge of the court, hitting her head on a concrete slab. The blow led to bleeding in the brain. The blood clot was surgically removed shortly after Kayla arrived in the emergency department, but many months of hospitalization and rehabilitation passed before Kayla was discharged.

The week after she returned home, Kayla picked a fight with her husband and yelled, "You're killing me! Go to hell!" as she slammed the bedroom door. Her husband was shocked at such uncharacteristic behavior from someone who had once been quite gentle. Kayla rejected hugs from family and friends who came by to see how she was doing. She got upset if anyone touched her and at one point pushed her son away, saying, "Go away! I hate you!" Her family could not understand why Kayla, who had always been kind and circumspect in her speech, was behaving this way. Her husband wondered whether the brain injury might be the cause: "She has such a short fuse these days." When Kayla announced that she was going to give away the family's beloved dog simply because the dog was getting older, her husband contacted Kayla's doctor about his concerns.

Personality changes are not uncommon after brain injury. In fact, the most significant problem years after a brain injury may be such changes, including increased impulsivity.

Symptoms

A simple definition of impulsivity is acting on a whim or acting without thinking of the consequences. A person with impulsivity may blurt out comments or say or do something without weighing the impact of their words or action on others. They may criticize a family member, whereas before they would have been supportive or said nothing. They may become uncomfortably blunt and even verbally aggressive, like Kayla, in the above scenario.

Impulsivity can also manifest physically. The person with brain injury may be more easily upset and have a lower threshold for acting out physically. Before the brain injury it may have taken a lot to upset them, but after the injury, they may be constantly on edge and seemingly quick to lash out emotionally or physically. This major change can be surprising to caregivers and family members.

Impulsivity can have significant negative consequences. For example, impulsive sexually inappropriate behaviors in public can lead to legal attention, especially if directed at minors. The person living with brain injury may also be more likely to get into physical or verbal confrontations, indulging in their anger rather than appropriately weighing the risks and physical and legal consequences, as they would have before the injury.

Impulsive behavior can be hard to manage even among close family members and can erode support from family, as can be seen in Kayla's story. This behavior, in turn, can make it more difficult to achieve optimal recovery. This is especially true if the person is seeking supports from services and systems that are not specialized in supporting individuals living with brain injury. If Kayla and her husband sought help from a therapist for marital issues and didn't disclose her history of brain injury, the therapist might well assume Kayla was exhibiting signs and symptoms of a personality disorder. The eroding of clinical supports can result in premature discharge and little follow-up for individuals who have mental health or substance use–related disorders, magnifying the functional impact of their brain injury.

Impulsive behavior is often associated with frontal lobe injuries. The delicate location of the frontal lobes, near bony prominences of the skull, makes them particularly vulnerable to damage from violent impact. The orbitofrontal cortex, located right above the eyes, is associated with self-regulation. Self-regulation is one of our high-level adult thinking skills, allowing us to quickly weigh options for words and actions and respond according to one's best interest. The orbitofrontal cortex, the anterior temporal lobes, and limbic structures (particularly the amygdala) within the temporal lobes and their connections form a neural circuit that usually provides impulse control. For example, frontal lobe areas such as the orbitofrontal cortex regulate the limbic system (the emotional brain). (Many of these brain structures are illustrated in figures 2.1a and b.) When the frontal lobe is damaged, a minor provocation sometimes can lead to excessive emotional response and impulsive behavior.

Reactions that are really out of proportion to the circumstances can be puzzling and, in some instances, frightening. The frontal lobes and its associated circuits serve as the brake that helps to keep our emotions in control. They restrain the other parts of the brain, such as the amygdala, which gushes with emotions when stressed.

In some cases, impulsivity and other personality changes that arise after brain injury are a magnification of tendencies that existed before the injury. Perhaps the person with brain injury had been a bit impulsive. After the injury, the impulsivity may intensify, now causing distress and more serious consequences. Some have argued that people with impulsive personality traits may even be more likely to suffer a brain injury to begin with because they tend to take more risks and are thus more liable to hurt themselves. But sometimes these changes occur in people who had no such personality traits before the injury, as in the case of Phineas Gage (see the box).

Drinking alcohol and taking illicit or even some prescribed drugs are high-risk factors for sustaining a brain injury. Alcohol and drugs alone can make people more impulsive. Chronic or excessive use of these substances can affect the brain and lead to greater impulsivity. At the same time, these substances can make people more likely to sustain a brain injury, which can exacerbate the impulsivity further, leading to a vicious

The Puzzling Case of Phineas Gage

The effects of frontal lobe damage were famously noted back in
the nineteenth century, after an American railroad worker named
Phineas Gage was hurt. Gage sustained a traumatic brain injury
when a rod he was using to prepare a dynamite charge explod-
ed, piercing his frontal lobes. He survived his injury and recovered
remarkably well in most ways. However, it soon became apparent
that Gage's personality had radically changed. "Gage was no longer
Gage," noted a coworker. He now spoke impulsively, was coarse and
rude in his social interactions, and didn't much care how he treated others. To put it simply, he became a sociopath. Gage's case is
a well-known example of what frontal lobe damage can do; there
may be no obvious evidence of injury except for extreme behavioral
changes, such as impulsivity. People who have sustained damage to
the frontal lobes can have trouble keeping their impulses in check.
They may blurt out things they are thinking that they would have
kept to themselves before the brain injury.

cycle. People who sustain a brain injury, therefore, should not drink
alcohol or use drugs

Management

If you are concerned about impulsivity, either for yourself or for a person
you care for, seek professional help. Untreated or poorly managed
impulsivity has the potential to lead to unsafe or dangerous behaviors.
Contact your primary care physician or a mental health professional
regarding your concerns; they will be able to help or will make appropriate referrals. Impulsivity may also be associated with other medical
or emotional problems, so assessment by a professional is mandatory. In

addition, neuropsychological assessments can help your doctors understand the nature and severity of the impulsivity. Test results can help to
guide treatment, which is multipronged and includes a combination of
medications, behavioral strategies, and environmental adjustments.

Medication

Some medications may help to improve frontal lobe functioning and
thus decrease impulsivity. Doctors now frequently treat frontal lobe
damage with amantadine, an agent originally used to treat the flu and
later Parkinson's disease. It affects functioning of two neurotransmitters
in the brain, dopamine and glutamate. Other medications that help
impulsivity include selective serotonin reuptake inhibitors (SSRIs) such
as Lexapro (escitalopram) and Zoloft (sertraline). Tegretol (carbamazepine) is an antiseizure medicine that may also be helpful, as may Depakote (valproic acid).

Environmental and Behavioral Therapies and
Lifestyle Changes

Family members and caregivers of people with brain injury should
encourage behaviors that will help in brain recovery and decrease the
incidence of impulsivity. For example, it's helpful for the person with
brain injury to have a daily routine or a timetable for the day. The person
with brain injury should have a hand in shaping their routine and agree
on the structure for their day. If you need help setting up a daily structure, ask for help from your clinician or from a rehabilitation therapist
such as an occupational therapist.

Minimize provocation when possible. The threshold for responding
to a stimulus and controlling self-regulation may be lower in people
who have suffered a brain injury. Such a reduced tolerance level can lead
to impulsive behaviors. Although it may be impossible to eliminate all
provocation, make note and be aware of what people, comments, and

situations have already led to impulsive behavior. Keep alcohol out of the house and avoid stressful topics, especially when the person with brain injury appears to be less capable of self-regulation.

There are many strategies that can help improve or manage self-regulation. Breathing techniques associated with yoga, for example, can improve emotional regulation. Breathing techniques can increase body awareness and help an individual to hit the pause button. Deep-breathing exercises and guided meditation may also be helpful in improving self-regulation.

Imposing external structure to compensate for frontal lobe dysfunction can be beneficial for persons with brain injury. Try to reduce distractors in their environment (surround them with fewer things to get impulsive about) or post reminders of useful self-regulation strategies around the house where they will see them. Organizational aids such as calendars or schedule organizers may also be helpful so that the person with brain injury knows what to do next, affording them less time or opportunity to be impulsive. By addressing the issue of awareness, giving gentle feedback and redirections, and creating a structured environment, you will help the person begin to internalize the strategies and improve awareness, and the impulsive behavior will diminish.

Positive reinforcement works better for everyone, both children and adults. This holds true for individuals who have brain injury as well and tends to work much better than punishment for people with brain injury, so avoid threats and nagging. Modeling positive behavior by showing the person how to act appropriately is another way caregivers/support persons can help. Redirect the person when they act inappropriately. Plan ahead and develop simple "impulsive-alert!" signals such as showing a time-out sign or saying a certain phrase when the person with brain injury is getting impatient. Have the individual decide on what works and what does not work. One family member noted that when she finds her husband getting impatient or edgy, she tells him, "Ralph, it's time to take some deep breaths." She had already worked this out with her husband as a sign that he may be losing control and needs to calm down.

Good nutrition and adequate hydration are both important elements for successful recovery after brain injury. There is some scientific literature to suggest that omega-3 fatty acids (found in fish oil) may help with psychiatric conditions and may be helpful in brain injury as well. However, more clinical trials need to be done to determine its effectiveness and adverse effects.

In summary, brain injury can affect the frontal lobes and make a person vulnerable to impulsivity. People who have frontal lobe damage can behave quite differently than they did before the injury, or the injury can amplify preexisting traits. Caregivers and family members can strive to remember to recognize the neurological basis of such behavior change and support the person with brain injury as they learn and practice self-regulation skills. Seek help and guidance from a professional trained in the effects of brain injury, as impulsive behaviors (and situations in which they occur) can change from day to day.

Tips and tools on how to manage the symptoms discussed in this chapter appear in tables 17.1 and 17.2.

TABLE 17.1. TIPS AND TOOLS FOR COPING WITH IMPULSIVITY AFTER BRAIN INJURY	
Take a Time-Out	Take a time-out when you find yourself triggered or getting agitated.
	Don't let your emotions control you. Learn to control them.
Practice STOP	**S** – Stop the urge to act or say the first thing that comes to your mind.
	T – Think about other options.
	O – Options: think about what has worked well in the past.
	P – Prefer the option that has helped the best.

Table 17.1 continued on next page

Practice Deep Breathing	Learn deep-breathing techniques and use them when you have the sudden urge to do something that has had bad consequences in the past. Using these techniques may not come easily at first, but practice helps them become a habit.

TABLE 17.2. TIPS AND TOOLS FOR CARING FOR SOMEONE WITH IMPULSIVITY AFTER BRAIN INJURY

Reward, Model, Redirect	*Reward*: offer praise when something is done well.
	Model: model acceptable behavior.
	Redirect: distract with positive or more appropriate behavior when they are doing something that might negatively impact their relationships and safety.
Use Codes	Use codes or signals when you see the person becoming irritable or edgy. Set up these codes with them when they are calm and able to listen and participate.
Watch for Triggers	Be alert for triggers that lead to impulsivity and avoid, minimize, or remove them.
Develop a Behavioral Plan	Develop a behavioral plan with input and agreement from the person.
	Be clear about boundaries and limits.
	As a family, determine acceptable behavior versus inappropriate behavior.
	Some behavior may be inconvenient or embarrassing but otherwise safe. In these cases, tolerating the behavior may be the best approach.
Don't Blame	Don't blame yourself or the person with brain injury completely.
	The person may be acting out for any number of reasons that have nothing to do with you. When in doubt, get help from professionals or other family members.

It's Nothing Personal	Try not to take the hurtful things the person says personally, and do not accept them completely.
Take No Abuse	Don't allow yourself to be abused. You have to be clear on what you will tolerate and what you will not.

Take-Home Points

Personality changes such as impulsivity are not uncommon after brain injury.

At times, preexisting impulsivity is exacerbated by the injury.

Impulsivity is acting or speaking without consideration of the possible consequences and the impact one's words or behaviors may have on others.

Damage to the frontal lobes that help self-regulate our emotions can lead to impulsive behavior.

Chronic or excessive use of substances such as alcohol can affect the brain and lead to greater impulsivity. People who sustain a brain injury, therefore, should not drink alcohol or use illicit drugs.

Exercise

Hold your horses! And **respond**; don't **react**.

Reacting is a quick knee-jerk action without thinking or planning. When a person reacts, they say or do the first thing that comes to mind without pausing to consider the consequences. Very often, reacting does not end well, either for the person who does it or for those around them. You only want to react when there is an immediate threat or danger, as the primary goal then is your safety. Otherwise, do not react—respond!

Responding is having a well-thought-out reaction. Response

has far better outcomes. So let's go over the steps to take when you are triggered or have an urge to act out:

• Pause. Do not say or do anything.

• Soothe yourself. Move to a calm place. Or do something calming such as taking deep breaths—take a few breaths until you feel really calm.

• Sleep on it. If you have to provide an answer or find a solution, take your time. If pressed, you can always say, "Let me think it over, and I'll get back to you." Take guidance from a person you trust or your health care professional.

Chapter 18

Substance Use

Billy, 32 years old, was making a left turn and did not notice a car coming toward him at a high rate of speed. He could not speed up quickly enough to avoid the other car, and it rammed him. He found his car spinning out of control and hitting the curb. He was dazed and disoriented as the paramedics arrived. At the hospital he was diagnosed with a mild traumatic brain injury. He did not have to be hospitalized, but he found himself with constant neck and back pain. To alleviate the pain, he was given a prescription for opioids. At first, he took them as directed to help manage his pain. Over time, though, he felt he needed more and more opioids to get through the day. His doctors, concerned about potential misuse of the prescription opioids, were not willing to provide refills. So Billy started buying opioids illegally. When he took them, his pain was better, but more than that, he found that he could forget his problems for a while. He also started to use alcohol in addition to the opioids, which helped numb his memories of the accident. Eventually, his use of substances caused major problems with his wife and family, as he was not participating in family activities and was frequently missing work. In addition, his wife noticed a change in his mood: he was more irritable and easily angered. Finally, his wife gave him an ultimatum—get treatment for substance use or they would have to separate. Billy, however, did not think he had a problem, continued to use opioids and alcohol, and refused to get treatment, until he was terminated at work for missing days. He then entered an outpatient substance abuse program and joined a 12-step addiction program.

Symptoms

Brain injuries can lead to increased use of substances such as alcohol, marijuana, opioids (painkillers), or street drugs. Usually there is a honeymoon period soon after the injury when people stop using illicit drugs or alcohol. This can last anywhere from a few weeks to a couple of months. After the honeymoon period, the risk of returning to pre-injury substance use levels increases. In a significant minority, in about 10 to 20 percent of cases, alcohol or illicit drug use may be a new problem following the injury.

There are many reasons why persons with brain injury use alcohol or illicit substances. This may be related to their pre-injury problematic use, an (unhealthy) coping strategy to deal with their traumatic experience, mood problems, pain, or increasing impulse control problems following the injury. Unfortunately, the use of these substances generally makes things worse, and there are many adverse effects of substance abuse, especially after brain injury. Brain recovery can be slowed down, and additional brain damage can occur within the context of substance use. Increased substance use can also lead to difficulty in maintaining structure in the day, which makes it harder for recovery to occur. Substance use can worsen certain problems following brain injury, such as cognitive issues, balance and gait, or emotional problems, and can also place individuals at risk for seizures. In addition, it can lead to disagreements with family or friends, potentially leading to less support at a time when greater support is needed. There is also research suggesting that people with brain injuries who use substances are at higher risk of being unemployed, living alone, or engaging in criminal activities.

Biology: Brain Regions Involved

Substance use often starts with an impulsive decision, even outside the context of brain injury, but as we discussed in chapter 17, brain injury may make impulsivity worse. Making an impulsive decision to use a substance may be driven by boredom, peer pressure, or a need to escape from everyday life stressors. Dopamine is a neurotransmitter that may play a large role in this sort of decision-making. It is important in what can be called the brain's "Want" system or reward pathway (which includes the ventral tegmental area in the brainstem and the nucleus accumbens in the basal ganglia, as well as connections to the amygdala, hippocampus, and the prefrontal cortex). This "Want" system signals what the brain wants to feel good. Substances can significantly increase dopamine in the "Want" system, leading to increased excitement and attention to and anticipation of reward. The reward itself is through the "Like" system (which involves the nucleus accumbens and the ventral pallidum), with release of endorphins and cannabinoids, as well as a chemical called anandamide (*anand* is the Sanskrit word for bliss).

The "Want" system includes the prefrontal cortex, which can modulate or inhibit excessive wanting. Unfortunately, with brain injury, this is one of the areas that are commonly damaged (especially in traumatic brain injury). Such damage can lead to lack of inhibition of the "Want" system, leading to excessive wanting. In the context of using a substance, the person with brain injury may find themselves wanting more than those without a brain injury, thus making it more difficult to control substance use.

Unfortunately, with continued substance use, many people will go from impulsive to compulsive use, whereby the use of the substances makes the brain's response to the substances change. The "Want" system can become more sensitive, leading to a compulsive level of wanting the substance. At the same time, the "Like" system can become less sensitive. Tolerance can build up, so that more of the substance is needed to get the same pleasure compared to before. Wanting can become greater, while liking can decrease, meaning that a person who is using substances has greater desire to use, but with less pleasure with each use. This pattern can lead to an addictive cycle, with cues or thoughts leading to a great drive to get the substance, only to have the actual substance use lead to diminishing pleasurable returns.

With the case at the beginning of the chapter, Billy's use of opioids exceeded the prescribed dose in his attempt to manage pain and stress, eventually leading to misuse, until he had difficulty keeping his job and managing relationships with family and friends. It is as if his brain had been hijacked and he was compelled to use more and more. This is, in fact, what substances can do: they are attractive at first by causing activation of the reward pathways in the brain (therefore it feels good), but activation of those pathways only leads to a dependence on the substance in order to maintain the reward, which comes at a cost (such as job loss, family disruption, loss of friends).

Management

Management of substance use disorders includes a comprehensive medical evaluation to determine the nature and severity of the substance abuse problem, triggers associated with use, medical/psychiatric problems present before and following the injury, the person's family and living conditions, and the strength of the person's support system. Based on this information, the doctor will make a determination on the type of treatment that is best suited for the individual.

Management of substance use disorders may include admission to a substance use rehabilitation facility or admission to an outpatient program, outpatient therapy, or medications. Therapy is predominantly focused on changing the behaviors of the person to stop or minimize use of substances and learning healthy coping skills to deal with triggers and stress that precipitate the urge to use. A simple behavioral approach could be to avoid situations, people, and locations that trigger want of the substance. Cues to use can be certain situations or certain locations where someone used in the past and are now associated by the brain with a memory of pleasurable use. Behavioral change could also involve replacing the substance use with a different behavior, such as exercise.

Medications can be useful to decrease activation of the reward system when the substance is used. For example, one FDA-approved medication for alcohol use disorder is naltrexone. Naltrexone blocks opiate receptors in the reward pathways in the brain, leading to less pleasure when using alcohol, thereby decreasing the positive effects of alcohol.

There can be withdrawal effects with substances such as alcohol, where neurons are now hypersensitive to alcohol and hyperexcitable. When alcohol intake stops suddenly, these neurons can trigger excessive activity and withdrawal symptoms (including potentially seizures) can occur. Acamprosate, another FDA-approved medication for alcohol use disorder, may help desensitize these hyperexcitable neurons to alcohol and restore the normal state of excitability, reducing the risk of relapse.

Ultimately, most successful substance use disorder treatment programs may use both behavioral and medication approaches. Programs often also target depression or anxiety disorders that may be contributing to unhealthy substance use. Family therapy, individual therapy, and group therapy are often helpful. Clearly, individuals living with problematic substance use often benefit from multiple modalities to help.

Tips and tools on how to manage the symptoms discussed in this chapter appear in tables 18.1 and 18.2.

TABLE 18.1. TIPS AND TOOLS FOR MANAGING SUBSTANCE USE AFTER BRAIN INJURY

Ready, Steady, Go	*Ask yourself*:
	Are you **ready** to make the change?
	Why is it important to make the change?
	What have you lost during the time you were using substances?
	What can you gain by getting sober?
	Steady yourself with these responses—repeat, review, reframe to make sure that you are ready for the change.
	Go. Get help. Talk to a person you trust and have them help you or find professional help.
Identify Your Triggers	What are your triggers—loneliness, boredom, anger, shame, guilt, pleasure?
	Or just an impulse?
	Whatever they are, they can be controlled.
	Write them down and talk to a professional counselor on how to control them—how to change the urge to use into a behavior that is comforting, soothing, or relaxing.
Go to Group Meetings	Make attending substance abuse meetings a priority.
	Try to attend meetings consistently and regularly.
	Meetings can help improve your knowledge, increase your support network, and teach you coping skills. You may also be of help to someone else who is in the group—and that can be a boost to your self-esteem.
Relapse Is Not the End of Your Recovery Process	Relapses are common aspects of rehabilitation. It is not the end of your treatment.
	While you may be upset, you don't have to feel ashamed or guilty. Talk to your doctor/counselor about this, and they will help you get through.

TABLE 18.2. TIPS AND TOOLS FOR CARING FOR SOMEONE WITH SUBSTANCE USE AFTER BRAIN INJURY

Do Not Judge	If you really want to help your loved one, refrain from judging them.
	Listen to the person and observe their behaviors so that you get an understanding of their triggers.
	As the old adage goes, you can catch more flies with honey than with vinegar—be a support and an asset to the person.
	By making remarks on their behavior, you may actually be distancing yourself, as the person may perceive them as attacks and get defensive or feel isolated.
Get Help	You can't do it alone. You will have to get professional help.
	Only a professional can determine the best treatment options for the person.
Set Boundaries	Your love, support, empathy, and care are important and necessary, but at the same time, you will have to set boundaries.
	Be very clear with the person on unacceptable behaviors and the consequences of indulging in them. Write out these behaviors and their consequences in a plan.
	Follow through with the plan.
	Remember that your goal is to empower the person, not enable them.
Do Not Give Up	Substance use disorders can be a challenging illness to treat, more so in people with brain injury.
	Relapses are bound to happen.
	Consider a relapse as another opportunity to help.
	Do not give up, because if you do, you might be sending a message that you have lost faith in the person's ability to make a change.

Take-Home Points

Initially after the injury, substance use often stops. However, increased risk of use returns after the initial recovery period.

Use of substances after brain injury may reflect that pre-injury use continues to persist following the injury, or it may be a new problem after injury—or it may be secondary to co-occurring mood and anxiety problems.

Whatever the cause may be, help is available. Your doctor will be able to lay out a treatment plan that may include participation in a rehabilitation program, behavioral/talk therapy, or medications, depending on the presence of other co-occurring problems.

Exercise

• *Avoid situations, people, and locations that trigger want of the substance.*

• *Remove any type of drug paraphernalia from your home or any other place you go to frequently, as they can be triggers for use/ relapse.*

• *Find something healthy, pleasurable, and of interest to you to fill the time that was being spent on drug use. Replace the substance with something positive.*

Chapter 19

Apathy

Tony is a 64-year-old male who struggled with frequent and severe headaches for about three months. He consulted his doctor about this issue, and a medical evaluation revealed a brain tumor, which his doctor called a meningioma, a benign brain tumor arising from the outer coverings of the brain (the meninges). The meningioma was about 6 centimeters in size and was situated in the front part of the brain—the frontal lobe. Because of the size of the tumor and Tony's frequent headaches, his doctor recommended removal of the tumor. Tony consulted with an experienced neurosurgeon and underwent surgery. The neurosurgeon was able to remove most of the tumor. After that, Tony underwent a brief course of radiation therapy, which he tolerated fairly well. After completing radiation therapy, he had about nine months of intensive outpatient occupational and speech therapies. As Tony went through this process, the therapists noticed that he was just not interested in participating in therapy. And even when he did, he would not push himself to complete the activities or would do just some of the activities at his own slow pace. His therapist described him as having "no initiation or motivation" to participate in therapy. He also appeared disengaged and uninterested in everyday activities. His wife worried, concerned that this attitude could not be healthy for Tony's brain recovery. She wondered how much of this behavior was just his being lazy and how much was due to the brain injury: "He's just a couch potato these days. He doesn't do anything!"

After much prodding from his wife, Tony agreed to see his primary care doctor. His doctor noted that he was awake and alert, and his physical examination was normal. When his doctor questioned him about his mood state, Tony replied that he wasn't sad or depressed; he just felt "dull." His wife added that Tony was eating and sleeping well, and he never once reported feeling hopeless or a burden to her. He was not using alcohol or drugs. Tony's primary care doctor referred him to a neuropsychiatrist with expertise in brain injury. After detailed evaluation, the neuropsychiatrist determined that Tony was suffering from a lack of motivation related to damage to the frontal region of his brain from the tumor and subsequent radiation, and diagnosed him with apathy syndrome.

Motivation is a murky concept, but we all intuitively have a sense of what it is. We can think of motivation as the ability to set a goal and take steps to achieve that goal. Typically, the things we are interested in are the things that motivate us. Other motivators might be the need to feed our families, pride in our work, or religious or ideological beliefs. Motivation is what gets us up in the morning, spurs us to do the many things we do in a typical day, and pushes us to persevere despite the inevitable setbacks in our days and our lives. Lack of motivation, interest, or concern is known as apathy.

Symptoms

The person with brain injury does not typically complain of feeling apathy. Rather, it is the person's caregivers or family members who typically notice the behavior. Perhaps they see that the person with brain injury does not finish tasks during rehabilitation or at home and has great difficulty completing tasks they have committed to. They may make plans for the next day but do not follow through, so plans never come to fruition. The person with brain injury may not commit to any goals at all. They may seem perfectly content just "being" and not particularly interested in "doing." Family members may complain that their loved one is "being lazy" or is a "couch potato" or that they do not "sparkle" anymore. They may think the person's personality has changed—no longer the vivacious, fun-loving, interested person they have known for so long. The person is now pleasant enough but flat.

The loss or diminished motivation can either be a problem with initiation (not starting a conversation, not seeking out social activities) or a problem with responsiveness (not feeling happy when good things happen or not feeling sad when bad things happen). Furthermore, it can affect any one or more of the domains of cognition, emotion, or behavior.

Apathy after brain injury is a common cause of conflict between the person with injury experiencing apathy and their family or caregivers. The family may feel that the person is not putting forth full effort and may become frustrated with them. They may feel that they are putting in hard work on the person's behalf, while the person has become lazy and is doing very little. They may feel that the person with brain injury is wasting the significant expense of rehabilitation therapy.

Apathy is often a direct consequence of the brain injury, but it can also be due to other medical problems. Apathy may be one of the symptoms of other psychiatric or other medical disorders or occur as an isolated entity (figure 19.1). Thyroid problems, infection, anemia, low testosterone, Parkinson's disease, Alzheimer's disease, vitamin deficiency, sleep problems, and environmental factors, among others, can all cause symptoms of apathy. Blood tests can rule out thyroid problems, vitamin deficiencies, anemia, and infection, so ask the doctor whether blood testing would be appropriate.

Consider not only general medical causes but also illicit drug use and medications as causes of apathy. Marijuana, alcohol, and narcotic pain medications are associated with apathy. Even selective serotonin reuptake inhibitors (SSRIs) and similar agents used to treat depression and anxiety can, in some people, cause apathy.

It is sometimes difficult to distinguish between apathy and depres-

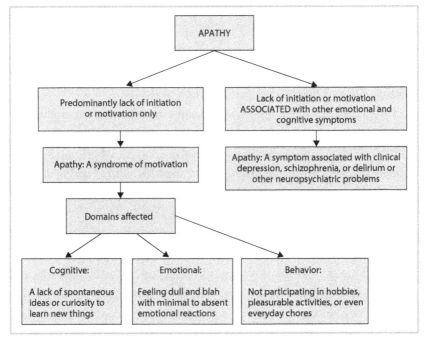

Figure 19.1. Different Aspects of Apathy

sion. Tony, in our opening story, for example, had symptoms predominantly of apathy, not symptoms of depression, such as sadness, feelings of hopelessness or guilt, or changes in sleep or appetite.

Of course, it is possible for a person with brain injury to have both apathy and depression. Apathy can be part of depression, but it is not always present in people who have depression. Conversely, depression can, but does not always, occur along with apathy. One way to distinguish between the two is to note that the core issues with major depression are lack of enjoyment and persistent low mood. The depressed person typically has poor self-esteem and little self-regard. The depressed person may also report feelings of hopelessness or suicidal thoughts or both. In contrast, the person with apathy may not feel or appear particularly sad. Persons with apathy may deny that they can't enjoy things; they are simply not interested in initiating or engaging in activities that could lead to enjoyment. In fact, they may be quite content doing nothing.

It is important to distinguish apathy from depression, not only to make an accurate diagnosis, but also because treatment can be different. As noted above, some antidepressants such as high doses of SSRIs can actually make people apathetic, so it's best to avoid certain antidepressants if the issue is truly one of apathy. On the other hand, some antidepressants do help apathy, so talk with the doctor to determine which antidepressant—if any—is best for the person with apathy. Some antidepressants are helpful for people who may have both apathy and depression.

To accurately diagnose apathy, the doctor will do a comprehensive evaluation. Typically, the doctor will ask the caregiver pointed questions about how the person with brain injury is doing. Be as open and honest as you can in answering these questions because your responses will help the doctor make an accurate diagnosis.

Apathy following brain injury is associated with less recovery and less response to treatment. This outcome is not surprising, given that a person with brain injury who is not an active participant in occupational, physical, or speech therapy is likely to make only limited progress.

Apathy can also magnify the functional impact of other common brain injury–related functional challenges such as poor attention, concentration, and memory. In addition, if the apathy is not understood to be directly related to damage to an individual's brain, it can be misinterpreted by those around the individual as laziness or selfishness. Unfortunately, the longer apathy goes undiagnosed and untreated, as discussed below, the more it can erode the person's support system, leaving them isolated and open to development of more behavioral health challenges.

Factors Associated with the Development of Apathy

Often apathy results from direct trauma to circuits in subcortical areas deep within the brain, including the thalamus, amygdala, and basal ganglia. A part of the basal ganglia called the ventral striatum is particularly important in our ability to sense pleasure and be motivated to act so that we achieve pleasure (this is part of the reward pathway, discussed in chapter 18). Interactions between these areas and the prefrontal cortex (especially the dorsolateral prefrontal cortex) and the medial prefrontal cortex and anterior cingulate lead to motivation. Damage to these areas and circuits can lead to apathy. In our case at the beginning of the chapter, the tumor was situated on the frontal lobe; the pressure caused by the tumor, the surgery, and the radiation therapy could have all contributed to damage or dysfunction of the white matter tracts connecting these subcortical structures to the frontal lobe, and this damage could have led to disruption of the motivation circuitry.

Management

Scientists believe that, at a neurochemical level, dopamine is an important contributor to motivation. The release of dopamine associated with something in our environment appears to make that stimulus more relevant, or salient, to us. In other words, dopamine allows the brain to tell itself, so to speak, that something out there is important. Dopamine prods our brains to engage in action. Perhaps not coincidentally, dopamine is involved in the control of movements. Increasing dopamine can thus increase motivation. Scientists believe that dopamine is critical for the "Want" system of the brain, the circuit of the brain that drives our wants, housed primarily in the ventral striatum in the basal ganglia. Medications that are predominantly stimulating and increase dopamine are used in the treatment of apathy.

Medication

Medications that increase dopamine include bromocriptine and stimulants such as Ritalin (methylphenidate) and Adderall (dextroamphetamine). These medications are used to treat apathy and seem to help some people, but they have not been adequately studied to determine that they are indeed beneficial. Amantadine, which indirectly affects dopamine, can also be used to treat apathy, but it too has not been adequately studied. Some doctors prescribe certain antidepressants to treat apathy, including Effexor (venlafaxine), Pristiq (desvenlafaxine), and Wellbutrin (bupropion). Other agents to consider include Sinemet (carbidopa-levodopa) and Eldepryl (selegiline). Finally, a class of medications called acetylcholinesterase inhibitors (which increase acetylcholine), which includes medications like Aricept (donepezil), Exelon (rivastigmine), and Razadyne (galantamine), can help with apathy in dementia and so may be helpful in brain injury as well. All of these medications, however, can have serious side effects, such as changes in heart rate or blood pressure, confusion, or delirium if taken in inappropriate dosage and without regular supervision by a physician.

Environmental and Behavioral Therapies and Lifestyle Changes

Behavioral and environmental methods are very important in the treatment of apathy. We recommend trying environmental and behavioral methods first, before using medications, because they have no side effects. If other possible causes of apathy (narcotic pain medications; high doses of SSRIs; alcohol, marijuana, or illicit drugs; medical disorders) are eliminated or addressed and apathy does not resolve, then a helpful approach may be to have the person with brain injury work with a professional, such as an occupational therapist (OT), speech-language pathologist (SLP), or rehabilitation neuropsychologist, to learn how to structure their days. Examples include mapping out a timetable for every day of the week that includes set times to do routine activities (bathing or taking meals, for example), enjoyable activities, exercise, and rest; establishing sleep time and wake time, and making to-do lists based on priorities. It is also helpful to build in rewards that the person can earn for following the timetable or completing tasks. Verbal cues (that is, telling the person with apathy what to do and patiently reminding them) may be helpful. Problem-solving training by an occupational therapist or a psychotherapist may also be helpful. Music therapy and singing can help. Having more stimulation in the environment can be helpful as well.

In summary, apathy is not uncommon after brain injury. Apathy is lack of motivation that can affect a person emotionally (making them feel dull, for example), behaviorally (causing trouble initiating and keeping up with tasks), and cognitively (slowing the processing of information). Apathy can occur with or without depression. Apathy after brain injury can be a major contributor to poor recovery. Family and caregivers must recognize apathy as a symptom of brain injury and be aware that the person with brain injury may be apathetic as a direct or indirect result of the brain injury. People who were not apathetic before their injury are unlikely to become less active just because they are just being lazy or resistant. Once you remember that fact, you can help the person with apathy receive appropriate treatment and help them through their recovery.

Tips and tools on how to manage the symptoms discussed in this chapter appear in tables 19.1 and 19.2.

TABLE 19.1. TIPS AND TOOLS FOR COPING WITH LACK OF MOTIVATION AFTER BRAIN INJURY: THINK APATHY

Activities	Think of activities you like to do. Start by doing simple, previously pleasurable activities.
Prepare	Make preparations and plan the day; make a timetable or schedule for the day.
	Remember the saying "By failing to prepare, you are preparing to fail."
Awake, Arise, and Act	You have to get off the couch or bed and do something. The longer you sit on the couch, the duller you will feel.
Team	Have a team—one or more people you trust who can serve as your external motivators.
Healthy Lifestyle	Think about what you can do to stay healthy. Make changes. Challenge yourself to do things differently.

| **You** | Go with whatever you want to do—your low-hanging fruit. It does not matter if it will lead to something or bring success. Doing something is better than not doing anything. This can serve as a springboard for doing other things later on. |

TABLE 19.2. TIPS AND TOOLS FOR CARING FOR SOMEONE WITH APATHY AFTER BRAIN INJURY

Avoid Labels	Do not blame the person or use labels such as lazy or couch potato.
Educate Yourself	Apathy is not laziness. It is not an intentional disengagement or defiance. Try to take a responsive as opposed to a reactive stance when interacting with the person.
Get Involved	Do not ignore the low-hanging fruit—help the person start with tasks that are easy and doable so that a sense of accomplishment is gained. Use external motivators such as reminders and model the behavior. Focus on collaborating rather than tutoring.
Request a Referral	If appropriate for the person with brain injury, request a referral to an occupational therapist or speech-language therapist who can work with them to plan and structure their days.
Avoid Drugs	Certain drugs and medications can cause or worsen apathy and are best avoided. If concerned about the person's drug use or medications, discuss your worries with them and their doctor.

Take-Home Points

Apathy is a decrease in or lack of motivation, interests, or engagement, and is not uncommon after brain injury.

Apathy after brain injury can be a major contributor to poor recovery and therefore diagnosis and treatment is important.

Exercise

• *Buddy up: find someone you can connect with to work, play, or get things done. This person can serve as your engine—your drive. Your buddy can also be your alter ego. Do something with this person (such as taking a new class, learning an instrument, traveling to a new place)—whatever you've always wanted to do but never had the initiative to do.*

• *Keep an activity journal. Every day, write down the activities that you did. It can be anything ranging from simple, basic activities to more complex things. This can serve as a stepping stone and launching pad as you work on your recovery.*

Chapter 20

Sleep

Laura, 16, slipped and fell when she tried roller skating for the first time and suffered a moderate brain injury when her head hit the curb. She has been sleeping poorly since she left the hospital. She falls asleep easily but has trouble sleeping through the night. She wakes up early in the morning, long before she has to, and has trouble getting back to sleep before her alarm goes off. When her doctor asked about other problems, Laura admitted she wasn't enjoying things the way she used to and just wasn't motivated to do much. She also noted that it didn't take much to make her burst into tears.

Dean, 44, suffered a severe brain injury when a tornado drove a tree through his front door, knocking him over as he ran for cover. He was in the hospital for three weeks, and then moved to rehabilitation. Bleeding in the brain and brain swelling complicated his medical recovery. Part of his treatment involved taking steroids, and since the brain injury, he has gained about 30 pounds. Now that he is back at home, he feels tired all day. He has also noticed that it is much harder for him to concentrate. His wife adds that Dean "snores like a freight train" and that his loud snoring keeps her awake at night.

Melanie, 35, sustained a brain injury after she slipped in the bathroom and hit her head against the sink. Now she can't get to sleep until two in the morning and repeatedly sleeps through her alarm, waking up around ten o'clock. This insomnia has been frustrating for her because she has to report for work by eight.

Symptoms

Sleep is an essential part of life. We all know this intuitively, as we often "don't feel right" or feel slower when we haven't had a good night's sleep. We feel tired or irritable. Words may not come to us as easily as when we need them in conversation. In fact, even though scientists are not certain about the exact functions of sleep, we do know that lack of sleep interferes with emotional stability, cognitive functioning, and social and functional productivity. Healthy human beings spend about one-third of their lives in sleep, demonstrating just how important sleep must be for normal body and brain functioning.

An injury to the brain can affect sleep. Sleep problems are about three times more common in people with brain injury than they are in the general population. In fact, more than half of people with brain injury experience sleep problems at some point during recovery. Undiagnosed or untreated sleep problems can make irritability, anxiety, depression, and memory and concentration problems worse and can greatly interfere with productivity and rehabilitation. The latter is important because engagement in rehabilitation is an active process that requires the person with brain injury to put forth a lot of time and energy to derive the most benefit from treatment.

Several regions distributed throughout the brain control sleep. Small groups of nerve cells maintain sleep (in the hypothalamus, particularly an area called the ventrolateral preoptic—VLPO—nucleus in the anterior hypothalamus) and wakefulness (in the basal forebrain, posterior hypothalamus, and nuclei in the midbrain and pons) and connect to other regions of the brain via complex circuits. There are many types of sleep disorders, and many have overlapping symptoms. Here we discuss only the most common sleep disorders and provide basic principles for diagnosing and treating them.

Sleep problems can occur without other symptoms or can be associated with other medical conditions, such as infections or depression. They are often associated with pain and fatigue, which many people with brain injury also experience. And sleep problems can affect people with brain injury regardless of how severe the injury is and can occur at any point during recovery.

The Stages of Sleep

Sleep is an active brain process consisting of two basic states: rapid eye movement (REM) sleep and non–rapid eye movement (NREM) sleep. NREM sleep consists of four stages, each of which lasts between 5 and 15 minutes. In normal sleep, we go through five sleep stages that can be differentiated by the electrical brain waves they produce, which differ in amplitude (size) and frequency (number per second). These five stages combined last a total of 90 to 100 minutes. People progress through a few such cycles during every normal sleep period. We recognize that shift workers often get their restorative sleep during daylight hours, but for the purposes of this discussion we use "a good night's sleep" and similar terminology to refer to a standard episode of seven or eight hours of sleep.

Sleep thus consists of alternating stages of NREM and REM sleep. NREM sleep predominates in the early part of the night. Four or five REM periods occur in a given night's sleep, each period longer than the previous one. REM sleep accounts for about a quarter of the total sleep time; in other words, we spend about two hours per night in REM sleep.

A structure at the base of the brain called the pons activates REM sleep. The pons relays signals to the thalamus, which screens the signals and then sends them to the cortex (the outer layer of the brain, responsible for thinking and planning).

The pons also sends signals to the spinal cord that temporarily paralyze the muscles. In some ways, this paralysis is a protective strategy, which prevents us from moving our limbs and acting out our dreams. In some people, this suppression does not occur, and they act out during dreaming. For example, someone who is dreaming about being attacked may thrash his hands and legs and even get out of bed, boxing and punching his "attackers." Some people have even hurt themselves while dreaming. This type of abnormality is called REM sleep behavior disorder.

About three-quarters of the time that we are asleep, we are in NREM sleep. Deep NREM sleep occurs in the first part of the night. Structures in the hypothalamus control NREM sleep. Other regions, including the thalamus and the reticular activating system (RAS), are also involved.

Infants spend about half their sleeping time in REM sleep, whereas adults spend less than a quarter of total sleep time in REM. Also, as we age, the time spent in stages three and four of the NREM sleep declines. As a result, older adults have predominantly stages one and two of NREM sleep.

Causes of Sleep Disorders

Sleep problems can be the direct consequences of the brain injury itself or can result from environmental, physiological, or psychological factors. In traumatic brain injury (TBI), for example, the most common type of brain injury is diffuse axonal injury (affecting those nerve fibers that connect different parts of the brain), and because sleep is controlled by several regions throughout the brain, it is not surprising that sleep disturbance is a common consequence of brain injury. In addition, damage to the internal biological clock in the brain (the suprachiasmatic nucleus) that controls sleep and wakefulness can alter sleep timing. Brain injury may also affect regions of the brain that maintain breathing and muscles that keep airways open, resulting in sleep-disordered breathing, called apnea. Apnea is a marked slowing or temporary cessation of breathing, which significantly decreases the oxygen supply to the brain. Finally, chemicals in the brain that maintain sleep and wakefulness (including serotonin, norepinephrine, and acetylcholine) are also disturbed in brain injury and contribute to sleep-wake disturbances.

Environmental conditions such as noise, stimulation, and bright lights are often associated with sleep problems. There is a bidirectional relationship between sleep and such factors as stress, anxiety, and depression: sleep disturbance can both precipitate those conditions and result from them. Although alcohol can help people get to sleep, it interferes with staying asleep. Medical conditions that cause cardiac and respiratory symptoms can also cause sleep disturbances or make them worse. Many medications can interfere with the sleep-wake cycle. Most over-the-counter medications and sleep aids contain antihistamines, which cause drowsiness, but they also cause dry mouth, trouble urinating, and constipation. Because these side effects can be the source of distress, interfere with memory, and further worsen sleep, it is best to avoid these medications.

Common Sleep Disorders

Laura, Dean, and Melanie in our opening stories represent the most common types of sleep disturbances, but there are many others. All sleep disorders fall into one of four common categories: sleeplessness (insomnia), excessive daytime sleepiness, sleep-disordered breathing (sleep apnea), and sleep-timing disorders (circadian rhythm disorders).

Insomnia

Insomnia is the inability to fall asleep or stay asleep. It is categorized as early, middle, or late insomnia. Early insomnia is trouble getting to sleep, middle insomnia is waking up and not being able to go back to sleep easily, and late insomnia is waking up earlier than needed and not being able to go back to sleep. All three forms of insomnia may be present in the same person, and all interfere with productivity. Late insomnia is often associated with clinical or major depression. Some research suggests that insomnia is more common in the first few weeks after brain injury.

Laura, in one of our opening stories, has both middle and late insomnia. She also has symptoms of clinical depression (crying spells, lack of motivation, and lack of interest), so it is quite likely that the clinical depression is causing her to wake up too early in the morning. The depression could be related to environmental factors (the brain injury has severely impacted her life), genetic factors (a family history of depression), direct effects of the brain injury on chemicals that regulate mood, or any combination of these.

Daytime Sleepiness

Drowsiness during the day is also common after brain injury. A comprehensive evaluation and overnight sleep study (described below) can be helpful in distinguishing the different causes for this problem. A correct diagnosis is important because the treatment depends on the cause. Two common causes of daytime sleepiness are sleep apnea (discussed below) and narcolepsy. Narcolepsy is a condition in which the person experiences episodes of sudden and uncontrollable sleep. Although narcolepsy is typically a genetic condition (or is perhaps caused by infection), there are reports of narcolepsy after brain injury. Hypersomnia refers to excessive daytime sleepiness. This term is sometimes used as an umbrella term that includes all forms of excessive daytime sleepiness or to describe daytime drowsiness in the absence of sleep apnea or narcolepsy. A sleep specialist can diagnose all these conditions in a sleep laboratory.

Sleep Apnea

A condition of abnormal breathing, sleep apnea has three forms: obstructive, central, and mixed. With any of these types, brief pauses (up to 20 or 30 seconds) in breathing reduce the oxygen supply to the brain. The reduced oxygen leads to sudden and frequent awakening from sleep, which in turn results in daytime drowsiness. Obstructive and mixed sleep apneas also involve frequent and loud snoring, which can be bothersome and frustrating to the bed partner. Other common factors associated with sleep apnea include being overweight or obesity and a family history of apnea.

It is possible that Dean, in our opening stories, has sleep apnea. He is snoring loudly and has excessive daytime sleepiness. A sleep study would confirm or rule out this diagnosis. His weight gain could be the reason for his sleep apnea. He may have gained weight because of the steroid treatment for the brain injury or because he could not exercise, as he used to do, while he was recovering. The sleep apnea could also be related to direct effects of the brain injury, including damage to areas of the brain that regulate proper breathing during sleep. A sleep study will contribute to a proper diagnosis and thus to appropriate treatment.

Circadian Rhythm Disorders

Circadian rhythm disorders are sleep-timing disorders. We all have certain patterns to our sleep, which vary from person to person. A person's circadian rhythm reflects when that person is most awake and when they sleep. Circadian rhythm disorders are broadly categorized as either delayed sleep phase syndrome or advanced sleep phase syndrome. In both types of circadian rhythm disorder, the duration of sleep may not change, but the timing differs: going to sleep very late (delayed phase) or very early (advanced phase). People with advanced phase sleep disorder are sometimes called morning larks and people with delayed phase sleep disorder are sometimes called night owls.

Melanie, in our opening stories, is an example of someone with a circadian rhythm disorder, delayed sleep phase syndrome. She has a tendency to sleep late, but is still able to sleep eight hours, waking up around ten in the morning. The causes of circadian rhythm disorders could be brain injury disrupting the biological clock, the person's environment (for example, exposure to excessive stimulation or light at night), or genetic influences. Unfortunately, Melanie's work schedule requires her to get up early in the morning. In additional to getting traditional therapy for this condition, Melanie might consider changing to a job that would allow her to start work later in the day.

Other Sleep Disorders

Other types of sleep problems include periodic limb movement disorder. Leg movements during sleep are not unusual, but uncontrollable and involuntary leg movements during sleep are often problematic. Restless legs syndrome (RLS) is a condition of painful creeping, crawling sensations in the legs that occurs when the person is lying down. These sensations interfere with sleep at night and cause drowsiness and fatigue during the day. Iron deficiency anemia and chronic renal failure can worsen RLS. Sleepwalking, as the name suggests, is walking or moving around during sleep or even doing some activity (eating or sitting up in bed, for example) while being unaware of doing so.

Diagnosis

Physicians who have expertise in sleep disorders are most qualified to diagnose a sleep disorder. Diagnosis usually requires a clinical evaluation and an overnight sleep test called polysomnography (PSG). Evaluations that include PSG or some other sleep study usually take place at night, but they can be performed during the day for people with circadian rhythm disorders or narcolepsy and for shift workers. In PSG, a technician applies electrodes to different parts of the patient's head and body. The electrodes feed into a central box, which in turn connects to a computer that records and stores the data. PSG measures not only electrical activity in the brain during sleep but also eye and body movements. PSG also records the duration of sleep, number of awakenings, and periods of REM and NREM sleep, all of which contribute to the diagnosis of conditions such as sleep apnea, narcolepsy, periodic leg movements, or RLS.

Management

The initial step in the treatment of sleep disorders is a comprehensive evaluation by a physician, which includes obtaining a medical and psychiatric history, reviewing medications, and reviewing the person's daytime schedule and bedtime routine. The doctor may also order an overnight sleep test to obtain objective data regarding the nature of the sleep disturbance. Based on all these results, the doctor will create a specific treatment plan.

Treatment of sleep disturbances depends on the cause. However, whatever the cause of sleep disturbance may be, sleep hygiene (see exercise below) is an important aspect of treatment. In addition, cognitive behavioral therapy for insomnia (CBT-I) has also been recommended as the first-line treatment for insomnia. Table 20.1 describes the different components of CBT-I.

TABLE 20.1. COGNITIVE BEHAVIORAL THERAPY FOR INSOMNIA AFTER BRAIN INJURY	
Relaxation Training	Use muscular relaxation, yoga, and meditation to reduce arousal and decrease anxiety.
Cognitive Therapy	Employ talk therapy to dispel unrealistic and exaggerated notions about sleep.
Sleep Restriction	Decrease time in bed to equal time actually asleep, and increase as sleep efficiency improves.
Stimulus Control	Strengthen bed and bedroom as sleep stimuli. Associate bedroom solely with sleep/intimacy.

There are multiple treatment strategies for managing several of the common disorders of sleep that can be associated with injury to the brain.

Mood or Emotional Issues
If sleep disturbance is secondary to depression or other psychiatric disorders, evaluation and follow-up with a psychiatrist will be necessary, as treatment should focus on medications and psychotherapy appropriate for that disorder.

Sleep Apnea
Primary treatment strategies include losing weight and quitting smoking. If either of these fails, the doctor may recommend using a device that opens the airway, called a continuous positive airway pressure (CPAP) machine. If you are concerned about sleep apnea for yourself or the person you are caring for, make an appointment with a specialist in sleep medicine, who can do the evaluation and provide treatment.

Circadian Rhythm Disorders

Exposure to bright light during strategic times during the day for specific periods helps restore circadian rhythms and promote sleep. Bright-light therapy uses a special light box that produces more light than indoor lighting. To be effective, the intensity of bright light should be about 10,000 lux (a measurement of light intensity). Bright-light therapy in the evenings is useful for advanced sleep phase syndrome and in the mornings for delayed sleep phase syndrome. Individuals differ, and bright-light therapy should be individualized too. There are many types of light therapy, and inappropriate exposure to light can have negative consequences. Therefore, light therapy should be done under the guidance of a knowledgeable health professional.

Melatonin is a natural hormone that controls our sleep-wake cycles. A doctor may recommend an appropriate dosage of melatonin to help the person fall asleep earlier. Clinicians who can evaluate and treat circadian rhythm disorders include primary care doctors, psychiatrists, neurologists, psychologists, and behavioral therapists with expertise in sleep disorders.

Medication

If the doctor is not able to identify a primary cause of sleep disturbance, he or she can recommend medications that can help with sleep. The doctor will choose medications based on the person's medical and psychiatric history. The medication should help the person sleep but not cause daytime sedation, cognitive problems, or behavioral side effects. It is best to avoid medications if possible, and to focus instead on sleep hygiene.

However, medications may be necessary in some cases. A sleep specialist is the best person to recommend medications to treat sleep disorders. But even when medications are recommended, they should be used for the shortest time possible, not more than a few days to a couple of weeks. Avoid using benzodiazepines, like Xanax (alprazolam), Klonopin (clonazepam), Valium (diazepam), or Ativan (lorazepam) to help with sleep. People taking such drugs regularly can build up a tolerance to them, and they can be addictive. Even long-term use of non-benzo-diazepine medications such as Ambien (zolpidem) or Lunesta (eszopi-clone) can cause daytime drowsiness, fatigue, and loss of coordination; therefore, long-term use is typically not recommended.

Environmental and Behavioral Therapies and Lifestyle Changes

Treating sleep disturbances always includes making environmental modifications and lifestyle changes. Non-medication strategies include practicing sleep hygiene, muscle relaxation, deep-breathing techniques, imagery, and cognitive therapy (which aims to substitute realistic thoughts for inappropriate thoughts and beliefs that contribute to sleep-lessness). It is best to work with a professional therapist who will be able to advise and guide you on the use of non-medication treatment strategies.

As a caregiver, if your sleep partner with brain injury is gasping for air while sleeping, it is important to consider an assessment for sleep apnea. Sometimes repositioning your sleep partner can help, or if you have a bed that can change the angle of the bed, doing so might be helpful. You can also remind your sleep partner not to exercise or eat right before sleeping, and you can help monitor the temperature of the bedroom to keep it cool when it is time to sleep.

In summary, proper sleep may be a big factor in successful recovery from brain injury. Caregivers of people with brain injury must understand just how critical sleep is to recovery and well-being. Unfortunately, the brain injury itself or factors related to the brain injury can make sleep worse. As we have discussed in this chapter, structuring the environ-ment to be more conducive to sleep is an important first step. If that is not enough, work with the doctor treating the person with brain injury to identify the underlying cause or causes of the sleep disturbance, which could be many things: anxious or depressive thoughts keeping the person with brain injury awake, medications the person is taking, new-onset narcolepsy or sleep apnea, disrupted normal sleep habits, or a number of other factors.

TAKE-HOME POINTS

Sleep problems are very common after brain injury.

Common types of sleep problems include insomnia, daytime sleepiness, sleep apnea, and circadian rhythm disorders.

Undiagnosed or untreated sleep problems can exacerbate emotional and cognitive problems and interfere with productivity and rehabilitation.

A comprehensive neuropsychiatric assessment is the first step, since management depends on the type of sleep problems.

In general, non-medication strategies such as environmental and lifestyle changes, as well as cognitive behavioral therapy for insomnia (CBT-I), should be considered first line agents.

Exercise

Sleep Hygiene

• *Maintain structure during the day. Try to establish a routine or a timetable, which helps sleep get regulated. People with brain injury, in particular, may need to set an even more rigid schedule, one that sets a specific time for getting up and going to bed every day.*

• *Get involved in hobbies and pleasurable activities. Engage in outdoor activities, as exposure to natural sunlight is important for maintenance of wakefulness.*

• *Exercise regularly. Do strenuous exercises such as jogging or aerobics in the morning and light exercises such as stretching or yoga during the evening. It is best to avoid exercising a few hours before you would like to sleep.*

• *Avoid daytime naps. If you must nap, limit your nap to no more than twenty to thirty minutes and try to do this around the same time every day. In other words, put the nap time on your time-table.*

• *Maintain a comfortable ambience in your bedroom. Set a temperature you are comfortable with. Cooler temperatures are better for sleep. Minimize noise and light.*

• *Avoid coffee, tobacco, or any other stimulants after noon.*

• *Use the bed only for sleep and physical intimacy. Avoid other activities, such as reading, talking, watching TV, or using electronic devices such as tablets or cell phones while you are in bed. The mere fact of doing these activities in bed can disrupt sleep. What's more, the background light of electronic devices can make sleep more difficult to achieve.*

• *Keep your bedroom stress-free. Don't use your bed as an office. Avoid working on the computer or laptop, paying bills, or doing job-related paperwork.*

• *Have dinner at least two hours before bedtime. A late dinner can lead to acid reflux, which can affect sleep.*

• *Avoid over-the-counter sleep medicines or any other non-prescription medicines.*

• *Avoid alcohol and illicit drugs. Although alcohol may help you fall asleep, it may inhibit your ability to stay asleep or to sleep well. It's best to avoid alcohol or illicit drugs while trying to overcome sleep disturbance.*

• *Don't watch the clock. Turn your alarm clock around when you are trying to sleep. Checking your cell phone or looking at the clock to see what time it is when you're trying to fall asleep can make you more anxious and make it harder to sleep.*

• *If you can't fall asleep within a reasonable amount of time in bed, get up, go to another room, and do something boring until you feel sleepy. Then go back to bed and try to sleep. If you still can't sleep after a reasonable time, then leave the room again and repeat the process. Do this as many times as necessary until you fall asleep. You want your mind to associate the bed with sleeping, not with not sleeping. The greater percentage of time that you are sleeping while in bed, the easier it will be to get to sleep when in bed.*

• *Consult a specialist. If sleep problems persist, have your doctor refer you to a physician with expertise in sleep disorders; a thorough evaluation, including sleep studies, can help in establishing the diagnosis. The diagnosis will determine the appropriate treatment.*

Part V

Cognitive Issues
Caused *by the*
Traumatized Brain

Cognitive issues can linger after brain injury, especially in people who have experienced a moderate to severe brain injury. Cognitive issues can affect our ability to think, remember, and plan; our ability to work and function independently; and abilities that are critical to our sense of self, of who we are, and how others see us.

Cognition is multifaceted and includes attention, memory, and other higher-order functions. We focus on discussing cognitive issues after moderate to severe brain injury. Persons with mild brain injury often have cognitive problems in the first few weeks after injury, but the majority of them make a good recovery within months. However, a small number can have persistent cognitive problems, typically associated with factors such as poor sleep, issues of adjustment, clinical depression, stress relating to ongoing legal issues, or factors outside the injury itself. Repetitive mild injuries (which we discuss in chapter 30) may also lead to cognitive issues.

We open the cognitive section of this book with attention problems (chapter 21) occurring after brain injury because we consider attention the foundation to other cognitive functions. We then discuss memory (chapter 22), executive function (chapter 23), and language (chapter 24).

Chapter 21

Attention

Michael is a busy 65-year-old lawyer with his own law practice in a small town on Lake Erie. After he sustained a right brain stroke, he was admitted to a stroke unit for a few days and then underwent inpatient and outpatient rehabilitation. By three months, except for some lingering left-sided weakness, he had recovered fairly well and returned to work. Michael had always prided himself on his ability to multitask and get things done—his practice and his clients depended on it. Now, several months after the stroke, he admits that he feels a lot slower; he reluctantly turned over two big cases to his law partner because he feared he wouldn't perform well in court. These days he keeps his office door closed so that he can really concentrate; he finds it supremely hard to focus when there are distractions in the hallway and outer office. "Any little noise bothers me. I just can't focus," he says.

Attention is a commonly used word whose meaning we all intuitively understand. In a more scientific sense, attention involves the ability to focus and choose something from a number of stimuli. At some point, we have all been told or told others to "pay attention." Without paying attention, we cannot learn or manipulate information or reach our goals.

Despite our intuitive sense of its meaning, attention is not one single phenomenon. There are three distinct forms of attention: selective attention, sustained attention, and divided attention. On a more fundamental level, we can think of arousal, the state of wakefulness that allows us to interact with the environment—as a form of attention, too.

How Brain Injury Affects Attention

The person with brain injury can experience a range of arousal states, from coma to hyperarousal (agitation). Impaired arousal generally occurs immediately after the brain injury, and the person becomes more alert as they gradually recover. People with brain injury can have problems with one or several subtypes of attention, from problems with arousal alone or compounded by deficits in selective, sustained, or divided attention (figure 21.1).

As people with brain injury recover, they may pass through a phase of delirium, which could be considered an attention disorder. People in a state of delirium cannot focus or sustain their attention for significant periods. Confusion and disorientation in this state can trigger agitation or even aggression. Although the delirium eventually lifts, difficulties with selective attention and sustained attention can persist for many people.

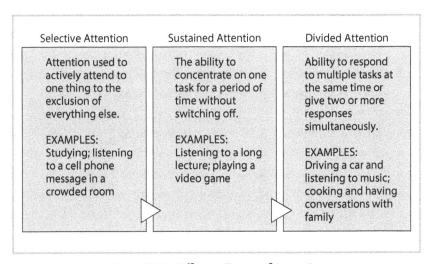

Figure 21.1. Different Types of Attention

Selective attention is the mechanism by which the brain chooses which stimuli in the environment to engage with. It involves the ability to inhibit or ignore the processing of distractions. When we think about paying attention or being distracted, we are usually referring to selective attention.

Sustained attention or vigilance refers to maintaining focus on something for a longer time than is required for selective attention. People who have experienced a brain injury may have trouble keeping their focus for more than a brief period, perhaps just seconds. As recovery occurs, both selective and sustained attentions tend to improve. Selective and sustained attention impairments usually occur in moderate to severe brain injury.

Divided attention is the ability to maintain focus on more than one task at a time. It reflects an ability to supervise aspects of attention because it involves switching between tasks. Divided attention is one component of executive function (see chapter 23). Divided attention difficulties can occur at all severities of brain injury. People with even mild brain injury can feel subjectively that they can no longer multitask efficiently. Fortunately, within the context of a mild injury, once factors such as life stress and poor sleep resolve, attention improves in many.

Attention is critical for other cognitive functions because we need attention to store things in memory. Once in memory, we can manipulate information and act on our goals. Because attention is such a basic and critical function, it depends upon diffuse neural circuits throughout the brain—and that arrangement is both good and bad. The built-in redundancy makes attention more resilient than other cognitive functions and therefore more quickly recoverable. On the other hand, because the circuits controlling attention are spread throughout the brain, a wide range of brain injuries can have an impact on attention.

Arousal, our baseline attention level, is housed in the brainstem, which connects the spinal cord to the rest of the brain. The reticular formation is the circuit in the brainstem that is critical in maintaining our ability to attend at all and that controls arousal. Damage to the reticular formation can result in coma. Without baseline attention, no other cognitive processes can be executed properly.

Selective attention involves a diffuse circuit that includes the posterior parietal lobe, the dorsolateral prefrontal cortex, and the anterior cingulate, along with the thalamus and basal ganglia. The thalamus, basal ganglia, and parietal lobe supply different types of input to the rest of the selective attention circuit, and in doing so, guide the targets of attention. For example, the thalamus sends sensory information, the basal ganglia sends motor information, and the parietal lobe sends spatial information throughout the circuit. Such input is vital because the selective attentional circuit needs to know where the sensory stimulus is that we have to attend to, and then where the target is that we have to respond to by moving our limbs. The dorsolateral prefrontal cortex and anterior cingulate are thought to utilize all this information to ultimately do the "selecting" of selective attention—that is, selecting to attend to something. (These parts of the brain are illustrated in figures 2.1a and b.)

Sustained attention, or vigilance, may involve the right hemisphere of the brain, particularly the frontal and parietal cortices. Divided attention may be related to other, even more diffuse, networks controlled by the white matter tracts connecting different parts of the brain.

Management

As with other types of brain injury, impaired attention is generally treated with a combination of therapies.

Environmental and Behavioral Therapies and Lifestyle Changes

Impaired attention benefits from both environmental and behavioral interventions. As a caregiver or family member of a person living with a brain injury, you can help by eliminating sources of distraction, particularly overstimulation. Because a person with impaired attention has trouble distinguishing between what they should pay attention to and what they should not, they may get overwhelmed and fatigued if there are too many people or too many things going on around them. Their inability to process overstimulation can also lead to irritability and agitation.

The person with brain injury who has attention problems can benefit greatly from having a predictable schedule. Plan activities that require significant attention and effort for times when they are rested. Sleep is thus a particularly critical factor in recovery. A person with brain injury who is not sleeping well will likely have trouble focusing their attention. (See chapter 20 for information about sleep disturbances and treatment.)

Cognitive rehabilitation is a formal approach to teaching cognitive skills and providing exercises to practice them. Attention training immediately after the brain injury is usually unnecessary because in most cases attention improves spontaneously as the brain recovers. During rehabilitation, however, whether in the rehabilitation hospital or at home, attention training can be helpful, and is best done with supervision and guidance from a clinician such as a neuropsychologist, an occupational therapist, or a speech-language therapist. Computer-based attention-training programs may be useful, although they are best done in conjunction with a knowledgeable clinician and may have limited generalization, meaning that improvement in attention scores on cognitive testing may not necessarily translate to improvement in activities of everyday functioning.

In addition, people like Michael in our opening story may benefit from learning compensation strategies working with a rehabilitation psychologist or a neuropsychologist, as well as collaborating with a vocational rehabilitation program, which can provide a range of services, ranging from job analysis and career counseling to case management and psychosocial interventions, thus helping people return to either their pre-injury work or find and obtain a new job. Supported employment once someone has returned to work is a critical support for many after a brain injury. The employment specialist can help the person transfer strategies and accommodations for brain injury–related challenges and offer feedback regarding work performance, relationships with employers and coworkers, and problem solving around such work-related issues such as transportation and ongoing health and medical needs. Supported employment is an evidence-based practice for successful reentry or entry (in the case of those injured at a young age) into the workplace.

Medication

Medications may also play a role in treating attention deficits after brain injury. They should be used only as prescribed by a doctor; self-adjustment or self-prescription can be dangerous and harmful, because these medications can lead to unwanted changes in heart rate or blood pressure.

Amantadine, an agent that acts on glutamate and dopamine, may help recovery of arousal and therefore help with simple attention. Other helpful medications include agents that increase dopamine and norepinephrine (stimulants) and agents that increase acetylcholine. Stimulants like Ritalin (methylphenidate) and Adderall (dextroamphetamine) can help with various aspects of attention. They can support arousal and improve sustained attention. However, these medications can also exacerbate other symptoms such as anxiety, and therefore they need to be prescribed by a medical specialist who is well versed in the multiple components of brain injury.

There is some evidence that medications such as acetylcholinesterase inhibitors like Aricept (donepezil) can also help with attention. These agents, however, are not as specific to attention as are stimulants. Although they can help a range of cognitive difficulties, they may be particularly helpful in controlling divided attention, as opposed to selective or sustained attention.

In summary, attention is a critical aspect of cognition because it is the gateway to other cognitive functions. Because circuits throughout the brain control attention, brain injury frequently affects attention. While problems with attention usually resolve over time, some people continue to experience difficulty with attention, and awareness of strategies and how to implement them can minimize the negative impact of attention disorders.

Tips and tools on how to manage the symptoms discussed in this chapter appear in tables 21.1 and 21.2.

TABLE 21.1. TIPS AND TOOLS FOR COPING WITH ATTENTION PROBLEMS AFTER BRAIN INJURY

Establish Structure	Establish structure and routine for the day. Try to maintain the same routine.
Minimize Distraction	Simple things like turning off the radio while driving or switching off the TV while having a conversation cuts down on distractions immensely.
	Electronic devices like smartphones or tablets and social media networks can add exponentially to the attentional burden, so it's best to minimize their use.
	Avoid crowded places or places with a lot of stimuli such as noise, bright lights, and loud music, or go to such places during off hours.
Maintain Sleep Hygiene	Maintain adequate sleep to make sure you get enough rest. Lack of sleep, poor quality of sleep, or sleep disorders (see chapter 20) can be a major cause of attention problems after brain injury.

Table 21.1 continued on next page

Seek Accommodations   Consult your doctor if you are a student and are
                           having trouble keeping up with schoolwork or
                           meeting deadlines.

                           Your doctor can determine whether you will benefit
                           from certain accommodations at school.

                           If you are in a postsecondary educational setting,
                           almost all colleges and universities have an office
                           of student services that helps students identify and
                           obtain accommodations in the classroom such as
                           untimed testing and use of a note taker.

                           It is possible that you may have underlying ADHD
                           (attention-deficit/hyperactivity disorder) that
                           predates your injury and was not previously
                           diagnosed and has perhaps been made worse by
                           the brain injury.

                           Consider seeing a physician who specializes in
                           attentional disorders to look into this possibility.

Consider Brain-Training Computerized brain-training programs may be
                           helpful to leverage the brain's plasticity, which is its
                           ability to use new pathways after injury that can help
                           with attention.

                           Only use such programs under the supervision and
                           guidance of an experienced clinician.

                           To maximize recovery, follow these brain-training
                           programs regularly. Frequency and consistency
                           are key; doing the exercises just once in a while is
                           ineffective.

*Note: Any one of these strategies by itself may not work. A holistic approach that
combines a variety of strategies is often necessary.*

TABLE 21.2. TIPS AND TOOLS FOR CARING FOR SOMEONE WITH ATTENTION ISSUES AFTER BRAIN INJURY

Educate Yourself	Educate yourself about attention problems related to brain injury so that you feel more confident about helping.
	Ask a professional or the clinician taking care of your loved one about strategies and dos and don'ts.
Be an Ally	Work with the person with brain injury.
	Help them organize tasks.
	Help them break tasks into smaller bite-sized pieces and use a stepwise approach to get them done.
	Do not expect them to work through activities without any distractions.
	If they get distracted by a thought or have an impulse to work on a different activity, simply jot that down on paper so that they can work on it after the task at hand is completed.

Take-Home Points

Problems with attention can be difficulty in focusing, difficulty maintaining concentration, or difficulty paying attention to two or more tasks at the same time.

Attention is an important aspect of our functioning, because we need to be attentive to filter out irrelevant information and learn and store information important to us, so that we can use this information and act on our goals.

Minimizing distraction, having a structured daytime routine, identifying one or two goals for the day, and focusing on one task at a time are important strategies that can help to reduce inattentiveness.

Exercise

Use a **PLAN**.

Prioritize what needs to be done for the day.

Limit to one activity at a time.

Approach tasks in a step-by-step manner.

Noise, stimulation, and other distractions should be minimized.

Chapter 22

Memory

A car struck Roseanne's car from behind on an icy road, and Roseanne's head banged hard again her windshield as she slid into a snowbank. Roseanne sat in her front seat, disoriented, for about 20 minutes, until the ambulance arrived to take her to the nearest hospital. In the emergency department, doctors diagnosed Roseanne with traumatic brain injury from contusions in the right and left frontotemporal regions of the brain; in other words, she had multiple bruises on the front and sides of her brain. She was admitted to the hospital for observation and monitoring and discharged several days later.

Physically, Roseanne recovered quickly, but she noticed at once that things were harder to remember than they had been. In her first few months back at home, she misplaced her cell phone many times, left the tea kettle boiling on the stove, and had to look up her husband's work number every time she wanted to call him. A few months after the accident, she started to feel hurt that her sister hadn't called to check on her, until her husband reminded her that her sister had called twice in the past week. Over the next several months, Roseanne grew more and more frustrated at her inability to remember things. She tried making notes about what she had to do—doctor's appointment, shopping lists—but then she forgot about the notes: "I have to write notes all the time but then I forget where I put my notes!" After Roseanne missed a third follow-up appointment with her neurologist, the doctor began to suspect that his 55-year-old patient was having serious repercussions from the brain injury, and he called her husband, who brought her in the next day.

Memory problems develop in many people after brain injury. Although this chapter focuses on memory difficulties, memory problems often occur together with other cognitive deficits, particularly impaired attention. For example, if we are not able to pay attention to information, we are not likely to remember it. Also, considering that brain injury can be a diffuse process that can affect much of the brain (and the connections between different parts of the brain), memory problems may reflect damage to multiple parts of the brain, which means that multiple, distinct cognitive deficits occur together.

Memory is not a single, unitary cognitive function, despite our intuition that it is one thing. We have an intuitive sense of what memory is and what it is like not to remember, but in the brain, memory is housed in different neural circuits, and there are different types of memory.

Memory is a collection of processes that lead to learning and recalling information. There are two kinds of memory: explicit and implicit. Explicit memory is what we typically think of as memory—information we must consciously make an effort to remember—for example, remembering what someone told us a few minutes ago, what we ate for breakfast yesterday, or what movie we saw last week. Implicit memory is more subtle—it's information we remember without consciously trying to: how to walk, eat with a fork, or ride a bicycle.

Explicit memory, in turn, can be either episodic or semantic. Episodic memory remembers personal events, like what happened at work yesterday or who came by for dinner tonight. Semantic memory remembers facts we learned in the past—for example, cars have four tires, or the blue whale is the largest animal.

Episodic memory is most commonly affected after brain injury. In most cases, the more severe the brain injury, the worse the episodic memory. Damage to episodic memory is what most caregivers of people with brain injury notice and struggle with. A good example of having an episodic memory problem is Roseanne, in our opening story. She couldn't remember conversations she had had with family and colleagues, and she often forgot where she had left her cell phone.

A person with brain injury may forget within minutes what is told to them. It may seem that they are ignoring what you told them, but it could well be that they have a deficit in episodic memory and simply do not remember what you said. Episodic memory is also the type of memory most affected by Alzheimer's disease. Such individuals may learn new information but rapidly forget what they learned. Alzheimer's disease attacks areas of the brain that house episodic memory; brain injury may damage those same areas.

Brain injury does not appear to affect implicit memory and semantic memory as much as it affects episodic memory. Brain injury can affect other aspects of memory, such as working memory and metamemory. Working memory is the ability to remember things for a few seconds and then manipulate and use that information. You hear a phone number on the radio, you memorize it, and then you call the number using your cell phone—that's working memory. Metamemory is memory of memory, that is, awareness of one's own memory. Deficits in metamemory can lead people with brain injury to deny they have any memory problems at all, which can have a negative effect on engagement in rehabilitation and on well-meaning suggestions from family or caregivers.

As stated earlier, memory is closely tied to attention. To remember something, we first need to pay attention. Working memory is an extension of our attentional system, letting us pay attention long enough to put things into memory. Working memory allows us to keep something (an idea, an image, a telephone number) in our brain for a few seconds before the brain stores it in short-term memory (which lasts minutes). The brain then transfers short-term memory to long-term memory. Brain injury tends to impact working memory and short-term memory more than long-term memory.

To remember something, then, we have to pay attention (use working memory) long enough to store the information in short-term memory and then transfer the short-term memory into long-term storage. We then have to be able to retrieve the information from memory. Brain injury can affect all these aspects of memory, depending on where the damage is.

Memory assessment is an integral part of determining the severity of brain injury. In addition, understanding how an individual's memory is impacted by the injury can help determine how functioning in everyday situations may change. Post-traumatic amnesia (PTA) is the period after an injury when a person has trouble remembering new information. The longer the period of post-traumatic amnesia, the worse the brain injury is considered to be. PTA can occur even after a seemingly mild brain injury in which the person did not lose consciousness.

The neural circuitry of memory lies at least in part in two areas of the brain: the inner (medial) side of the temporal lobe, known as the hippocampus, and the upper outer surface of the frontal lobe, known as the dorsolateral prefrontal cortex. Unfortunately, the temporal and frontal lobes are both particularly vulnerable to brain trauma and are often damaged in brain injury.

The medial temporal lobe circuit is important in episodic, short-term memory; it stores information that we have just learned, perhaps what someone said to us a few minutes ago. Of course, for information to be learned (get into short-term memory), the attentional system (which has networks across much of the brain) must send the information to the memory system. The attentional system first sends the information to the working memory system, which is housed in the frontal lobe. The frontal lobe sends that information to the medial temporal lobe for short-term storage. Eventually, information from short-term memory is distributed to various locations throughout the brain for long-term storage. Visual long-term information goes to visual areas; long-term auditory memories go to auditory areas, and so on. The frontal lobe plays a critical role in organizing memories and permitting appropriate access and retrieval.

So, what seems like an automatic process—remembering what someone asked us to do a few minutes ago—involves the proper functioning of multiple areas of the brain. Normally, we do this quickly and automatically, but brain injury can cause difficulty at multiple steps of the process. The person with brain injury may have trouble with working memory, so they can't keep the information around long enough to store it. If they can store the information in short-term memory, they may have trouble organizing the information. Even if that mechanism is intact, they may not be able to retrieve the information quickly and accurately.

Management

How to manage memory problems after brain injury is dependent on many factors, including the severity of the injury, type of memory problems, and additional factors such as co-occurring medical and psychiatric problems. Assessment of memory problems is best done by a neuropsychologist with expertise in brain injury who conducts comprehensive pen and paper tests of memory and thinking to determine the severity and variety of cognitive deficits.

Treatment modalities are typically focused on remediation and compensation, though at times medication can be helpful. In cases of mild brain injury, long-term memory impairments are not anticipated. Although during the first days to weeks individuals can experience problems with memory, these difficulties usually improve with time. The key is adequate rest for the first week and then a gradual return to activities. Long-term rest after a concussion is no longer recommended and has been shown to have a potentially negative impact on quality of life. Education about the recovery process during the initial period following mild brain injury can help improve positive expectations of recovery. Most people with mild brain injury recover their memory capabilities spontaneously, without treatment or rehabilitation. Full recovery, as defined by the ability to organize new memories and retrieve them as efficiently as before, typically improves in days to weeks, but can take up to three months. It is also important to decrease the chances of a second brain injury. State concussion laws across the country provide guidance recommending that anyone who sustains a mild TBI while playing sports should come out of the game immediately, not returning to play until cleared by a medical professional. This advice is partly to avoid further brain injuries, which could complicate the recovery process.

Recognizing the problem is the first step in helping the person with a brain injury. Caregivers or family members may not realize that they are having difficulty learning and remembering new information and may blame them for not following instructions or for being careless. During rehabilitation, family and caregivers should work with the person with brain injury and memory problems to manage the person's expectations and advocate patience.

Environmental and Behavioral Therapies and Lifestyle Changes

At home, building structure into the day and minimizing distractions improves memory function. Avoiding overstimulation can help. Having a predictable schedule for sleeping, waking up, taking meals, working, and other activities can make more things automatic, so the brain doesn't have to work so hard. Protecting the brain from becoming overtaxed can in turn be helpful in recovery. Keeping things in the same place all the time can help the person with memory problems stop misplacing items. Repeating tasks in an organized way can help internalize the information and develop a habit. For example, keeping the keys in a particular place, such as on a table by the front door, can free up more brain bandwidth to take on new challenges. These steps maximize the chances of success and increase confidence for the person with brain injury.

Have the person with brain injury and memory problems do the most taxing tasks of the day at a time when they are most rested. Build rest breaks into the day to minimize fatigue as much as possible and maximize memory performance. Make visitors and guests aware that they should not disrupt the person's rest time or schedule.

Cognitive aids, such as notebooks, cell phones, tablets, calendars, and other devices, can cue memory. Not only can these items provide reminders when needed but, more importantly, they can also reassure the person, allowing them to worry less about having to remember. Relieving them of this responsibility lets them relax and, paradoxically, may help them remember better.

Cognitive rehabilitation with a brain injury professional focuses on strategies to improve memory or compensate for deficits and to set up the environment in ways that enhance memory performance. Cognitive rehabilitation services can be provided by speech-language therapists and occupational therapists, as well as psychologists, cognitive therapists, and other brain injury professionals. One of the challenges for the person with brain injury is to generalize what they learn in a formal cognitive rehabilitation setting to home. Therefore, the goals of rehabilitation are to learn to make things more automatic (by repeated behaviors), to strengthen previously learned patterns of behaviors, to learn compensatory strategies, and to generalize what they learn in the clinical setting to home and community, so that the person is able to have a better quality of life.

Medication

Medications to improve memory are a supplement to the techniques discussed above. However, in some cases they can be helpful, particularly in moderate to severe TBI. Two classes of medications may be helpful: those that increase the neurotransmitter acetylcholine and those that boost the effects of the neurotransmitters dopamine and norepinephrine.

Aricept (donepezil), Exelon (rivastigmine), and Razadyne (galantamine) are medications that increase acetylcholine. All three are also used to treat Alzheimer's disease. The research studies of the use of these medications in brain injury show mixed results, but in our experience these drugs may help improve memory in some people.

Agents that increase dopamine and norepinephrine can lead to cognitive improvements. They include Ritalin (methylphenidate) and Adderall (dextroamphetamine), agents often used to treat ADHD. An advantage of these medications is that they are quick-acting and may improve attention and processing speed and thus improve memory indirectly. Studies of these medications in persons with brain injury generally show some cognitive benefit.

Amantadine is a medication that was originally used to treat the flu and is still used occasionally to treat Parkinson's disease. It affects dopamine and another neurotransmitter, glutamate. Some studies indicate that amantadine may help with some cognitive processes, mostly attention, processing speed, and executive functioning. As we have discussed, these other cognitive functions may affect memory as well. Amantadine may thus indirectly improve memory. Namenda (memantine), a derivative of amantadine, is used to treat Alzheimer's disease and may enhance overall cognitive function.

Drugs that work primarily to increase dopamine, such as Sinemet (carbidopa/levodopa), Eldepryl (seligiline), and Parlodel (bromocriptine), may be helpful in some people with brain injury.

Certain antidepressants may also be helpful in treating memory problems, especially if there are also additional symptoms of clinical depression. However, the data supporting a benefit from these agents is weaker than for the mainstays of cognitive enhancement in brain injury: stimulants like Ritalin (methylphenidate) and agents that increase acetylcholine, like Aricept (donepezil).

In summary, memory is not one single process. There are subtypes of memory, and many other areas of cognition affect memory. Persons with brain injury and memory problems often become frustrated trying to remember things that were easy for them prior to the injury but are now a major struggle. Because our brains normally change all the time—in the process referred to as neuroplasticity—every time we learn something new, the capacity to recover is built in. Supporting the person with brain injury and memory problems as they go through rehabilitation, helping them structure their days, and encouraging them to follow their doctors' advice and take medications as prescribed will all help them greatly in their recovery.

Tips and tools on how to manage the symptoms discussed in this chapter appear in tables 22.1 and 22.2.

TABLE 22.1. TIPS AND TOOLS FOR COPING WITH MEMORY PROBLEMS AFTER BRAIN INJURY	
Embrace "A Place for Everything, and Everything in Its Place"	Make sure there is a place for everything, and keep things in the same place every time.
	Consistent organization like this may help you to stop misplacing items and can cut down on unnecessary frustration.
Use Memory Aids	Use external devices such as notebooks, cell phones, tablets, and calendars to make notes to help cue memory.
	Place sticky-note reminders throughout the house, especially in commonly used rooms like the kitchen, bedroom, family room, and bathroom, to help you remember tasks.
Get Help	If you are having difficulty working on a task because you cannot remember directions given to you, get help. In cases like this, teaming up with someone to do tasks can be enjoyable and lead to task completion.
Maintain a To-Do Board	Don't try to learn something new or master a new task in one go. Take breaks, practice, and try other strategies if the one you are using is not working.

TABLE 22.2. TIPS AND TOOLS FOR CARING FOR SOMEONE WITH MEMORY PROBLEMS AFTER BRAIN INJURY	
Avoid Practice Errors	As the person is learning a task, it is most beneficial to keep their mistakes to a minimum so they don't learn how to do a task incorrectly or inefficiently.
	Be clear and consistent, and repeat tasks and steps several times to minimize errors.
Be a Team Player	Support, guide, redirect, and assist, but do not overpower.
	Do not focus on "creating the building"; focus on "laying the bricks" regularly.
Consult If Concerned	Emotional well-being is an important aspect of learning and training. If concerned about the person's emotional health, consult a mental health professional.

Take-Home Points

Memory is not a single, unitary cognitive function; it is a collection of processes that lead to learning and recalling information.

What often seems like an automatic process—remembering what someone asked you to do a few minutes ago—actually involves the proper working of multiple areas of the brain, which can be damaged or dysfunctional in people with brain injury.

Having a structured routine, making environmental modifications (such as creating a safe place and having specific places for specific things), using memory aids (such as apps, sticky notes, calendars, or locator devices), and maintaining general wellness (taking care of emotional and physical health) are cornerstones of treatment.

Exercise

The Five **R**s to Cope with Memory Problems

• **R**ecite (if you have heard something) or read (if it is written information) or rearrange (if they are items in a specific place).

• **R**epeat—repeat to yourself the content—what you've heard, read, or rearranged.

• **R**eorganize the information. Examples: form a mnemonic; form an association by pairing it with something familiar; label items, doors, or cabinets; group items on shopping list into categories.

• **R**edefine and refine your skills by learning other strategies to compensate for your loss.

• **R**ehearse—rehearse and practice the reorganized information.

Chapter 23

Executive Function

Laura was diagnosed with a brain tumor and underwent surgery, radiation therapy, and chemotherapy. After about three months of treatment in the hospital, 47-year-old Laura was transferred to a recovery unit for intense rehabilitation. Despite weeks of arduous therapy and valiant effort, Laura was not permitted to return home after rehabilitation because she was unable to manage her own affairs. The occupational therapist (OT) evaluated Laura and declared it unsafe for her to live alone. In her report, the OT gave several examples to explain her decision: Laura could not follow the steps to write a check, pay bills online, or fill out a simple form, so she was incapable of managing paperwork or paying bills. And although Laura was physically capable of simple activities such as making a sandwich or peeling vegetables, she had difficulty staying on task—during the OT evaluation, she prepared an omelet but walked away without switching off the stove. Her medical team determined that Laura was clearly having executive function difficulties. They suggested that Laura and her family contact their local Aging and Disability Resource Center (ADRC) or local Center for Independent Living (CIL) or the Brain Injury Association of America (BIAA) to review what services and supports she might be eligible for so that she could be safe and independent within her home and community (options such as having supervision/assistance with an aide or supportive living environments were discussed).

Cognitive problems can occur following a brain injury, as we discuss in earlier chapters. As noted, there are several aspects of cognition, such as memory, attention, language, and executive function, and although we consider these functions separately, in reality there is a great deal of overlap among them. In this chapter, we focus on executive function.

Executive function is the ability to plan, organize, and sequence thoughts, plans, and actions to complete a task (to put toothpaste on a toothbrush, brush the teeth, and rinse the mouth to complete oral hygiene), monitor whether one's behavior is leading to its goal, and notice when mistakes are made and fix them. Executive function, in short, is the ability to set a goal, initiate action toward the goal, monitor progress toward the goal, and modify the course if necessary to achieve the goal.

Executive function strongly relies on prefrontal lobe functions—*pre* indicating the front portion of the frontal lobe. In persons with TBI specifically, the prefrontal lobes are particularly vulnerable to injury because the lower portions of the prefrontal lobe sit on the bony interior ridges of the skull and are thus likely to be injured in mechanical trauma to the head. Deficits in executive function are often a critical component in the level of functioning in a person with brain injury— for example, whether the person can live independently.

There are three aspects of executive function: cognitive, motivational, and emotional. From a cognitive point of view, executive function capabilities direct other cognitive functions, such as attention, memory, language, and movement. For example, the ability to pay attention to several things at once—such as taking care of the casserole in the oven while making a salad—depends on executive function circuitry in the brain. The executive function system has to allocate attentional resources, select an attentional target, deal with interfering information, and switch between things that need to be attended to. Working memory, the ability to manipulate information held in memory for a few seconds, is also an executive function, as is the ability to efficiently organize this information into long-term memory. As you can see, executive function can include and overlap with attention and memory aspects that are discussed in chapters 21 and 22.

Symptoms

A person with a brain injury who has problems with the cognitive aspects of executive function may appear to have problems with attention, memory, or reasoning. They may not speak as fluently as they did before the injury. They may take longer to think of the right word. Their thinking may be slower. Even if they can complete the task, it may take them longer to do so, and they must put more effort into it. Even a person with a mild brain injury during the first week can have noticeable problems in these areas, especially when they have to perform demanding or complex tasks, though for mild brain injury, these challenges will fully resolve over time unless other factors are impacting functioning (such as poor sleep).

Scientists believe that the cognitive aspects of executive function, such as working memory (the transient ability to hold, process, and manipulate information) and other higher-order functioning such as planning, organizing, decision-making, and problem solving, are associated with a part of the frontal lobe called the dorsolateral prefrontal cortex (the upper and outer part of the prefrontal cortex). Cognitive executive function can be impaired even without direct damage to the dorsolateral prefrontal cortex, but in such cases, the cause is usually damage to the white matter tracts that connect this part to other parts of the brain. Damage to these connecting tracts is common in brain injury (particularly TBI), even though the damage may not be evident on our usual MRI scans. Damage to the dorsolateral prefrontal cortex or the circuits arising from it can result in difficulty retrieving recently learned information, multitasking, planning complex tasks, filtering out irrelevant stimuli, and conceptualizing, organizing, and abstracting.

Another circuit, the ventral part of the prefrontal cortex (particularly the orbitofrontal cortex), lies at the border between the cognitive and emotional parts of the brain. At this strategic location, the orbitofrontal cortex integrates emotion with cognitive function. It is involved in guiding social behaviors and mediates self-monitoring and regulating behaviors within a social context. This part of the brain is particularly vulnerable to TBI, and damage to it likely explains the deficits in real-life decision-making and social functioning that are common in people with TBI. Damage to this part of the brain is associated with disinhibition, impulsivity, and socially inappropriate behaviors. People who have damage to the ventromedial prefrontal cortex, like Phineas Gage (see chapter 17), have trouble understanding others' feelings, being socially appropriate, and keeping their impulses in check. In other words, damage to the lower portion of the prefrontal lobe is associated with an increase in inappropriate social behaviors. Often, people with damage to this circuit may end up having conflicts with loved ones or in their interactions with people at work. Unfortunately, such behavior can lead to termination from jobs (even though they are capable of doing the work), since their behavior can be perceived by others to be rude and obnoxious.

Executive function circuits also include the medial prefrontal cortex (the middle portion of the prefrontal lobe), the part of the brain responsible for motivation: setting goals, initiating action, and sustaining activity until the goal is met. Significant damage to this circuit can result in diminished will to do anything. Thus, damage to the middle portion of the prefrontal lobe is associated with apathy (see chapter 19) or, simply put, "flatness." The term *abulia* is sometimes used to describe a moderately severe form of apathy.

Flatness refers to a lack of expression in response to a situation at hand. In one case, an individual with a significant brain injury to his medial frontal lobe was gently told of the violent deaths of two of his family members. His facial expression and his voice when reacting to this news would have been more appropriate for hearing the day's weather forecast. When people have difficulty matching their responses to the situation at hand, it can be very jarring to those around them and can lead, over time, to social isolation due to the lack of reciprocity during interpersonal exchanges. A more extreme form of apathy or abulia, in which the person may not move or speak, is called akinetic mutism. Typically, however, a person with abulia is slow to complete tasks, has a decreased ability to speak fluently, and has a hard time initiating or starting a task. Scientists believe that a particular part of the medial prefrontal cortex, the anterior cingulate, is important in these functions.

Thus, the medial prefrontal cortex helps in choosing a goal and initiating action, the dorsolateral prefrontal cortex is involved in planning and monitoring the action, and the orbitofrontal cortex integrates emotion with cognitive function.

We have discussed the three distinct aspects of executive function: cognitive, motivational, and emotional. But brain injury often causes diffuse damage that affects multiple aspects of all those circuits. Laura from our opening case, for example, had surgical removal of the tumor followed by radiation and chemotherapy, which probably caused diffuse brain damage. TBI is also a typical example of diffuse brain injury. It is helpful for you as a caregiver of a person with brain injury to be aware of these circuits and the behaviors that can stem from damage to these areas of the brain so that you can make sense of the behavior of the person with brain injury. The person may be slower to process information than before. They may have trouble solving simple, everyday problems. They may need help to organize and plan their day. They may act inappropriately in public. It's common for a person with brain injury to have a combination of some or all of these issues.

Management

There are things that you as a caregiver can do to help the person with brain injury who is living with executive function impairment. First, know that individuals typically do show some improvements over the first year/years. Nonetheless, residual difficulties are not uncommon, and it can be helpful to have reasonable expectations. The individual may appear slower or more disorganized or act differently post-injury. Treatment and consistent support and feedback can help increase awareness of executive functioning–related challenges, and over time, people can learn how to integrate strategies to diminish the impact on their lives and relationships.

Environmental and Behavioral Therapies and Lifestyle Changes

One woman who had a traumatic brain injury was very aware of her new situation: "I used to be the multitasking queen," she said, "but now I can only do one thing at a time." Because organizational skills are often impaired after brain injury, help the person to get organized and stay organized. For example, they may need help organizing their home office or keeping their calendar up to date. They may benefit from a regular schedule. Because they may have trouble planning and sequencing, help them to break small tasks down into smaller components and guide them on what to do next. Family members may need to assist with bill paying or other complex tasks until the person recovers.

Cognitive rehabilitation can help retrain the brain and teach skills to compensate for impairments in executive functioning. This type of teaching usually happens in a neurorehabilitation program staffed by rehabilitation neuropsychologists, physical therapists, speech-language therapists, and occupational therapists who are specially trained to work with people with brain injury.

Depending on the nature of the injury, one or more of these experts works with the person. Rehabilitation can involve collaborating with the person by role playing to teach ways to improve self-regulation and overcome obstacles.

A formalized neurorehabilitation approach to help with organization and executive dysfunction is known as Goal Management Training (GMT). GMT is a metacognitive training program to help people learn how to be self-aware of their thinking process, set task goals, complete tasks, assess performance, and extrapolate knowledge gained doing a particular task to use in other activities.

The training incudes education, mindfulness practice, and completion of assignments, with the goal of helping the person create goal-directed activities and carry them out successfully. The steps include identifying a task that needs to be done (setting a goal), developing a plan for attaining the goal, working through it by breaking it into small steps, rehearsing the steps if need be, completing the task, and analyzing the outcome. The results of the task can be used to formulate and complete another task. For example, if the goal is cleaning the house, the therapist works with the person on making smaller goals to attain the main goal of cleaning. They may first start by assessing the status of the house and then plan on cleaning different rooms on different days. The therapist rehearses with the person what needs to be done and how it is to be done, and the person starts with one room. Based on how this goes (the time taken, the effort needed, and the cleanliness of the room), they either keep the plan or revise it. The whole idea is to teach the person to be more organized, less distracted, and be able to successfully complete tasks.

Cognitive rehabilitation can also focus on retraining social skills that teach the person with brain injury what to do when they meet a stranger, for example. A person with brain injury who exhibits socially inappropriate behavior can benefit from consistent feedback about increased appropriate behaviors, redirections (pointing out the inappropriate behavior and redirecting them to other acceptable behaviors) and positive reinforcement (a reward or praise) when they act appropriately in a social situation. The goal of therapy is to help the person learn social skills at first in a structured clinic setting and then gradually help them to transition these skills to real-life settings.

Medication

Medications are not the primary method of treatment for people with executive dysfunction, but some medications are indeed effective, especially when executive function deficits overlap additional emotional issues such as depression or cognitive challenges such as inattention.

Amantadine affects several neurotransmitters, including glutamate and dopamine, and may help people with poor executive function after brain injury both cognitively and behaviorally. It may help to facilitate self-monitoring and hence improve behavior.

Acetylcholinesterase inhibitors like Aricept (donepezil) affect a neurotransmitter called acetylcholine and may help executive function in addition to their primary benefit of improving memory.

Stimulants like Ritalin (methylphenidate) and Adderall (dextroamphetamine), which affect dopamine and norepinephrine, may also be used. They clearly help with processing speed and attention, and they may improve the attentional aspects of executive function.

In summary, damage to executive function capabilities because of brain injury can cause significant functional impairment. These changes can be subtle, and it may not be apparent that they are due to brain damage. People may think that the person with brain injury is being stubborn or lazy or difficult. Caregivers who understand the aspects of executive dysfunction also understand that cognitive and behavioral changes after brain injury may reflect brain damage and may not be deliberate. Of course, it is important to help the person with brain injury regain a sense of control over their life. Encourage them to follow their doctors' advice and to actively participate in their rehabilitation. Discourage them from doing things that can make executive function worse, such as using drugs or alcohol or engaging in reckless behavior. With the support of family, people with brain injury can relearn skills and accept their new baseline while improving their lives.

Tips and tools on how to manage the symptoms discussed in this chapter appear in tables 23.1 and 23.2.

TABLE 23.1. TIPS AND TOOLS FOR COPING WITH EXECUTIVE FUNCTION PROBLEMS AFTER BRAIN INJURY

Don't Blame Yourself	If you are having difficulty getting motivated, don't blame yourself or label yourself as lazy or useless.
	Find an external motivator, since your internal motivation may not be working—like a family member, a friend, a coach, or anyone you trust who can give you a gentle nudge, or even use technology such as an alarm or alert system.
Work on Your Frustration	If you feel overwhelmed or have difficulty completing a task, first stop and take a break.
	When you feel calmer, write down the list of activities you have to do, from simple to more complicated, and set a goal of doing one or two tasks per day.
	If it is a complex task, write down the different steps of the task and follow them one by one.
Remember the Traffic Light	If you are having difficulty controlling your emotions or urges, come up with a stop-think-act mantra or a visual image (such as a traffic light: red = stop; yellow = think; green = go).
Know Your Strengths and Weaknesses	Do not indulge in behaviors that have the potential to worsen your thinking and mood. Examples include taking alcohol, illicit drugs, or even some over-the-counter medications.
	Focus on behaviors that have given you good results.
	Use similar strategies to do other tasks.

TABLE 23.2. TIPS AND TOOLS FOR CARING FOR SOMEONE WITH EXECUTIVE FUNCTION PROBLEMS AFTER BRAIN INJURY

Maintain Structure	Structure in all forms reduces both stress and disorganization. Keep a daily schedule, a routine, and a plan that the person with brain injury can count on to structure the day.
Maintain Consistency	Consistency promotes learning. Consistent responses to behavior and consistent daily routines, for example, will help the person with brain injury learn what is expected and what they can rely on.
Maintain a Schedule of Activities	Keeping a schedule for daytime activities that includes built-in breaks increases engagement and reduces boredom and fatigue.
Apply Rules, but with Flexibility	A code of conduct needs to be maintained for the person with brain injury, but it cannot be black-and-white—there must be opportunities for compromise. Behaviors that may appear odd or strange but are not harmful or unsafe are permissible. In other words, you don't have to fight every battle. Just fight the battles that are worth winning. You will find by using this approach that successes will build upon each other. Structure and consistency are important but remember that "genius has always allowed some leeway."
Practice Positive	You can catch more flies with honey than with vinegar.

Table 23.2 continued on next page

Reinforcement	Positive reinforcement in the form of reward or praise for good behavior encourages and thus helps maintain that behavior.
	Merely punishing the person for behavior they can't control can lead to outbursts and rebellious behavior. Redirect inappropriate behavior.
	Punishment never has any good effect.
Anticipate Stress	Write and rehearse scripts for coping with stressful situations.
	Work with the person with brain injury to practice what they will do in certain situations so that when the situation arises, the appropriate response comes easily.
Get Professional Help	If the person you care for is in trouble for acting out, work with professionals to explore options for helping them.
	Physicians, psychologists, and therapists may all be on the team that can help the person struggling with the executive function to manage.

TAKE-HOME POINTS

Problems with executive functions can interfere with school and work life, relationships, and even everyday activities.

Changes can sometimes be subtle and be misinterpreted as laziness or bad behavior.

It is important to help persons with brain injury regain a sense of control over their lives.

Encourage them to follow their clinicians' advice and to participate in rehabilitation.

Discourage them from doing things that can make executive function worse, such as using drugs or alcohol or engaging in reckless behavior.

With the support of family, people with brain injury can relearn skills and accept their new baseline.

Exercise

The Four **S**s to Cope with Executive Function Problems

• **S**afety: *Safety comes first. Whatever you are doing or dealing with, make sure it is safe. You have to protect yourself from injuries with complex activities such as driving.*

• **S**upport: *Surround yourself with people who love and care for you.*

• **S**trategies: *Work with your health care professional to learn healthy coping strategies.*

• **S**orry: *Don't hesitate to say you're sorry when you have offended someone. Letting go is always a good way to resolve an issue and move forward.*

Chapter 24

Language

At age 67, Nadira sustained a massive left-brain stroke, which left her with right-sided weakness and severe language problems. The language deficit was predominantly difficulty in producing words. She had difficulty speaking fluently and saying more than three or four words in a sentence; however, she could understand what was being told to her. With inpatient and later outpatient rehabilitation, the right-sided weakness improved, but her language continued to be a problem.

As months went by, Nadira felt fine physically, but her language difficulty, particularly with finding the right words and expressing herself, continued to persist and was very frustrating for her.

The medical name for disturbance of expression and comprehension of spoken language is *aphasia*. Aphasia may also be associated with deficits in written communication (dysgraphia) or reading (dyslexia). Language has a very specific circuit in the brain, and science is familiar with this language circuit and how it functions. People with brain injury can experience aphasia if the damage they suffer directly impacts the language circuit in the brain.

Symptoms

Aphasia has two fundamental forms: non-fluent aphasia (also known as expressive aphasia or Broca's aphasia) and fluent aphasia (also known as receptive aphasia or Wernicke's aphasia). People with non-fluent aphasia have difficulty speaking—much like what Nadira is experiencing. Their speech output is diminished or minimal—or nonexistent: some people become nonverbal. People with non-fluent aphasia may use only single words or short phrases. Speech is slow and effortful. Their speech may sound telegraphic, like an old-fashioned telegraph, composed of only a word and then a pause, a word and then a pause. As in a telegraph, only the main words in a sentence, the nouns and verbs, are used, without many words that connect them. Despite their trouble speaking, however, people with non-fluent aphasia generally remain able to comprehend speech. They can usually respond to verbal requests but cannot repeat phrases.

Fluent aphasia is characterized by deficits in understanding and comprehension. People with fluent aphasia use words that are incorrect for what they want to express. Such substitutions are called paraphasias. People with this condition are fluent, meaning that they speak at a normal rate and pronounce words correctly, but others have difficulty understanding them because what they say does not make sense. Fluent aphasia is sometimes also called jargon aphasia because of the odd substitutes people with this condition use for words: they say *car* when they want to say *far* or *cat* when they mean to say *dog*. Many people with fluent aphasia are frustrated that others cannot understand them, but they may lack insight into their own language dysfunction.

Anomia, or difficulty in naming objects, is a form of fluent aphasia and is a common language problem in people living with brain injury. A person with anomia might say, for example, that they wanted to get the cat out when they meant that they wanted to get the car out. The person with anomia may appear to have memory problems, but what is really happening is that they are unable to find the right word.

Some people have intact fluency and comprehension but have trouble repeating phrases. Damage resulting in both fluent and non-fluent aphasia can result in global or total aphasia.

Aprosody, another type of language problem seen in people with brain injury, is difficulty in appreciating or portraying emotions in speech. Much of what we communicate through our speech is more than just the words we speak, and much of the emotion we convey with our speech is not expressed in the words themselves. Being able to understand the emotions behind the words is an important human skill. But a person with aprosody may have difficulty understanding that when someone who is angry says, "Well, that's great!" they are being sarcastic. They may interpret the phrase literally and wonder why, in the midst of something going wrong, someone would say "that's great." In addition to difficulty in understanding the emotions associated with speech, they may also have difficulty modulating their speech and expressing their words with emotion. For example, their speech pattern may be monotonous and flat.

Understandably, then, aprosody as a consequence of brain injury can affect how a person living with brain injury interacts with their family and caregivers—a frustrating situation for all involved. For example, a newly married man whose brain injury leaves him unable to recognize emotions in his wife may not be able to comfort her when she is sad, or rejoice with her when she is happy, as he had before the injury. This scenario often leads spouses to tell rehabilitation professionals that "this isn't the person I married."

Language is one of the most localized and best understood cognitive functions in the brain. We know that the frontal and temporal lobes of the brain are associated with the ability to express, comprehend, and repeat, and we know that these lobes are associated with the ability to incorporate emotions into language. Although brain injury can cause diffuse damage, the frontal and temporal lobes are particularly vulnerable to traumatic injury, and left-brain strokes can commonly affect the frontal and temporal lobes, leading to language problems.

For most people, the left hemisphere of the brain houses language and is called the dominant hemisphere for language functions. This is always the case for right-handed people (most of the population), but the language circuitry of left-handed people tends to exist, to some degree, in both hemispheres—the left and the right.

Within the left dominant hemisphere, the language circuit includes

Wernicke's area, in the upper temporal lobe, which controls the comprehension of spoken and written speech; Broca's area, in the lower frontal lobe, which processes information into an organized pattern necessary for verbalization; and the arcuate fasciculus, which connects Wernicke's area and Broca's area. Damage to Wernicke's area can cause fluent aphasia; damage to Broca's area can cause non-fluent aphasia; and damage to the arcuate fasciculus can cause difficulty in repeating speech, or conduction aphasia. Anomia is common in brain injury because it results from damage to areas near Wernicke's area in the temporal lobe and the inferior parietal lobe. Anomia can also occur because of the more diffuse brain damage of the type commonly seen in TBI.

Other aspects of language involve different areas of the brain. The non-dominant hemisphere (the right side of the brain for most people) manages the "body language" and emotional content of speech. The non-dominant hemisphere is also responsible for cursing, likely because of the emotional aspect in cursing, so damage to the dominant hemisphere usually does not affect a person's ability to curse. It can be startling to hear someone who cannot speak more than a few words suddenly curse fluently! Finally, because singing can also reflect non-dominant hemisphere functioning, people with brain injury and non-fluent aphasia may not be able to engage in normal conversation but may retain the ability to sing what they want to express.

Management

Without an understanding of the subtleties of language dysfunction that can develop after brain injury, it is easy to misinterpret problems with language as lack of motivation and depression. Although the person with brain injury may be depressed—and that possibility certainly must be considered—it is also possible that they are having trouble expressing themselves well, so they may speak less than they did before the brain injury.

When the person with brain injury cannot seem to find the right word when they need it, they may get frustrated, and they may express their frustration as irritability or even agitation. As a caregiver, try to understand the reason for their irritability. Reassure them and provide them with a calm and soothing environment. Responding to their frustration with anger will likely agitate them even more and cause them to have more trouble expressing themselves.

Encourage the person with brain injury to put forth full effort in speech therapy. Being there for them during this intense therapy time, being patient with them as they relearn language skills, conversing with them, and exposing them to language can be very helpful.

Speech-Language Therapy

Treatment of language disorders caused by brain injury primarily involves speech and language therapy. Many people with brain injury improve their language substantially with aggressive therapy. Because in many cases people with brain injury have more subtle language disorders than classic fluent or non-fluent aphasia, often anomia or aprosody, working with a speech and language pathologist well versed in brain injury is critical in determining whether the person's cognitive problems are due to impairments in memory or language. These problems may be exaggerated by depression, anxiety, or other mood disorders; they will require the expertise of a health care professional, such as a neuropsychiatrist, neuropsychologist, neurologist, or a clinician familiar with brain injury, working alongside a speech and language pathologist. A neuropsychological assessment can also typically be helpful to tease apart the cognitive and emotional components of a person's presentation.

Speech therapists have various methods to help language recovery. For example, melodic intonation therapy (MIT) is sometimes used by speech therapists for people with expressive aphasia. The principle is that singing, rhythm, or intonation can stimulate the undamaged right hemisphere and help transfer of language function to the right side of the brain.

In the past, the accepted wisdom was that if language does not recover within six months, speech therapy should be discontinued. As we have learned more about the brain and its capacity for plasticity or adaptation, it has become clear that speech therapy is helpful for much longer than a few months after the injury. Although insurance coverage may be limited to a specific duration of time for therapy, longer and more extensive therapy is often useful in maximizing recovery. Practice at home, with family and friends, can be helpful as well.

Medication

The data on whether medications help language dysfunction after brain injury is limited. Cognitive enhancers including stimulants (such as Ritalin) or acetylcholinesterase inhibitors (such as Aricept) may help with cognition, but it is unclear whether they specifically help with language. These drugs may enhance cognition in general and improve language indirectly. Key elements to recovery are avoiding drugs and alcohol, maximizing social interaction, treating mood or anxiety problems, and engaging in speech therapy, with medication supplementation if needed.

In summary, language problems that develop after brain injury often include issues with expression, trouble comprehending spoken language, difficulty with both expression and comprehension, and difficulty naming items. All these forms of language dysfunction may be associated with a loss of rhythm and melody in speech. Conversely, a person with brain injury can lose melodic speech even though expression and comprehension are intact.

Tips and tools on how to manage the symptoms discussed in this chapter appear in tables 24.1 and 24.2.

TABLE 24.1. TIPS AND TOOLS FOR COPING WITH A LANGUAGE PROBLEM AFTER BRAIN INJURY

Get Professional Help	Consult a speech-language pathologist (SLP), also known as a speech therapist. SLPs can do many things to help the person with brain injury who has language problems.
	Make sure your SLP specializes in cognitive linguistic disorders and focuses on the language problems that commonly occur after a brain injury. An SLP who has experience with brain injury is usually the most suited to address cognitive linguistic disorders, not SLPs who address speech disorders such as stuttering or developmental problems.
Enhance Communication Strategies	Find a place that is quiet and calm. It can be difficult to communicate when there are distractions, noise, or other stimuli.
	Do not pretend to have understood when you have not.
	Do not hesitate to ask people to repeat what they said.
Keep It Simple	Think about the best way to communicate with people—simple writing, drawing, or use of picture boards can be helpful.
	Don't struggle to get it right or use words that are difficult for you.
	It is fine to substitute similar words for the ones you are trying to say.
	Use words or phrases that come easily to you.
	Some people find that using gestures or drawing the first letter of the elusive word with their finger helps them to come up with it.
Take Your Time	Make sure you have enough time for important conversations. If you are feeling fatigued or annoyed that the conversation is not going well, do not continue.
	Stop and take a break.
	Do not rush. Take your time.

TABLE 24.2. TIPS AND TOOLS FOR CARING FOR SOMEONE WITH A LANGUAGE PROBLEM AFTER BRAIN INJURY

Join the Team	You can support the person with language problems by attending therapy sessions and being an active member of the person's care team. You can work with them at home as they practice the strategies they have learned in therapy.
	During your practice sessions, ensure that the environment is calm and free from distractions.
	Try to make sure that the person isn't tired and is able to pay attention.
	Always remember that you are a family member first and an extension of rehabilitation therapies second.
Don't Shout	The person with brain injury may have language problems, but they are likely fully able to hear information. Loud talk can upset or worsen their frustration.
	State things clearly and keep your voice at your normal volume and your words at your normal rate of speech. Use words commonly used by the person before their brain injury.
Keep Communication Simple	Keep communication simple, but do not treat an adult with brain injury like a child.
	Try to maintain as normal a life as possible by including them in family conversations.
	If the person can understand what you are saying, you don't have to simplify.
	Do not overload the person with a lot of information.
	Do not focus on the person getting the words/sentences right. If you get the message they are trying to convey, that's success.
Get Professional Help	If you notice symptoms such as dips in mood, tearfulness, or lack of interest in someone you are caring for, tell their doctor about these changes.

Take-Home Points

There are two common forms of aphasia: non-fluent aphasia and fluent aphasia.

People with non-fluent aphasia have difficulty expressing themselves: they use only single words or short phrases. Speech is slow and effortful. They are able to comprehend speech, however.

People with fluent aphasia have difficulty comprehending speech but are able to speak fluently. However, they may use words that are incorrect or sometimes make up new words.

Difficulty naming, difficulty repeating, and difficulty appreciating or portraying emotions in speech are other types of language and communication problems after brain injury.

The recommended treatment is speech and language therapy, preferably by a speech-language pathologist with experience and expertise in brain injury.

Exercise

MIND your language.

• *Messages: Keep messages short and simple and use simple words.*

• *Invent: Be innovative and invent ways you would like to communicate such as gestures, simple writing, and drawing. Come up with signals for commonly used words—yes, no, thank you. Trying a picture board can also be helpful. A speech-language pathologist or rehabilitation neuropsychologist can help you come up with ideas for what might work best based on your strengths and weaknesses.*

• **N**oise: *Noise and distractions should be minimized when you are communicating.*

• **D**rift away from the topic if you want a break. Pausing, smiling, crying, or sighing are ways of communication too.

Part VI

Other Symptoms
of the Traumatized Brain

In this part, we discuss brain injury problems that do not fit neatly into mood, behavioral, or cognitive categories (but may have mood, behavioral, or cognitive consequences). These include headaches (chapter 25), seizures (chapter 26), visual problems (chapter 27), balance problems (chapter 28), and hormonal problems (chapter 29).

Chapter 25

Headaches

Ashley was a sophomore in college and a star on the school's diving team. At practice one morning, she miscalculated as she attempted to execute a complex dive. She hit her head on the diving board and splashed into the pool below, unconscious. Her coach pulled her from the water as other team members called for an ambulance. Ashley woke up to paramedics strapping her to a spinal board and carrying her out of the pool house. In the ambulance, she felt confused and disoriented, and she vomited during the short ride to the hospital. Emergency department staff took a CT scan of Ashley's head, and the results were normal. Doctors discharged Ashley that same day with the diagnosis of concussion.

Over the next two days, Ashley's confusion and tiredness improved, but she developed a severe headache. Her physician ordered another CT scan, and the results were again normal. Ashley continued to have headaches, which manifested in two forms: a dull pressure around her head, present most of the time, and worsening bouts of throbbing pain associated with vomiting and sensitivity to light. Her doctor advised her to get adequate rest, maintain a healthy lifestyle, and use Imitrex (sumatriptan) if necessary for her severe headaches. But the headaches persisted, and Ashley became frustrated and anxious. She wasn't sleeping, and she was falling behind at school. "My head hurts all the time," she said. Her productivity at home and school greatly declined and she went on a medical leave of absence. At six months after her injury, seeing no improvement, Ashley's parents consulted a psychiatrist at the recommendation of her primary care doctor, as they noticed Ashley was getting increasingly anxious and sleeping poorly. After evaluating Ashley, the psychiatrist prescribed Cymbalta (duloxetine) for the headache and anxiety symptoms and referred her to a therapist with expertise in mindfulness meditation, given the interrelationship between pain and mood. The combination of therapy and medications helped Ashley significantly, and she returned to school.

Headaches are a common complaint after brain injury, particularly after mild TBI. Severe TBIs can also lead to headaches, vomiting, and severe pain, especially immediately after impact. If vomiting and severe pain occur after a brain injury, seek medical attention immediately, because these symptoms can reflect increased pressure in the brain, which is dangerous because the hard skull drastically limits where the brain can go when it is under pressure. In the worst cases, increased pressure shifts the brain and traps the brainstem—the part of the brain that connects to the spinal cord—in the back of the head, which can be fatal.

In some people with brain injury, as times goes on, headaches can become a chronic problem. There are many types of chronic headache, and many factors can influence how chronic the headaches become and what symptoms occur with them. Depression, anxiety, post-traumatic

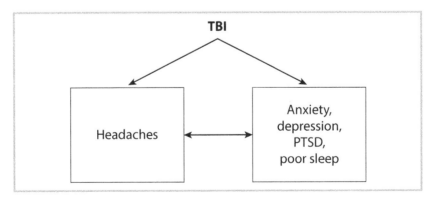

Figure 25.1. Relationship between Headaches, Mood, and Sleep after Traumatic Brain Injury

stress disorder, and sleep problems can all play a role and contribute to the chronic nature of the headaches and the intensity of the symptoms. The complex relationship between brain injury and headaches is depicted in figure 25.1.

Symptoms

Although headaches from a mild brain injury are generally less severe than those from a severe injury, they can nevertheless become persistent, and therefore very problematic. They can be triggered or worsened by light and sound sensitivity, and they can be associated with dizziness. Most headaches resolve within the first few days to weeks and almost all within the first few months, but in some cases they do persist.

The common forms of chronic headache that develop after brain injury are listed in table 25.1. Tension-type headaches are common after brain injury. These headaches often worsen as the day progresses. Tension-type headaches typically manifest as tightness in the neck and a feeling that there is a tight band around the head, but the person has little or no sensitivity to light or sound. These headaches often respond to Tylenol (acetaminophen) or Motrin (ibuprofen). In most cases, tension-type headaches do get better over time, but it may be worth consulting a headache specialist if these headaches persist for months. Non-medication techniques such as massage and stress management can help alleviate tension-type headaches and decrease their prevalence. It is also possible that overuse of medication is causing the headache: daily use of headache medications may, ironically, cause more headaches, a phenomenon known as rebound headaches. The headaches usually improve when the pain medications are stopped.

Headaches after brain injury can mimic migraine headaches. Migraines often involve significant sensitivity to light and sound, and people with migraines report pulsing and pounding of the head. When these kinds of headache occur, the person suffering will likely want to be in a quiet, darkened room. Of course, what triggers a migraine varies from person to person, but common triggers include stress, lack of sleep, irregular sleep schedule (getting too much sleep on the weekend and too little sleep during the week), caffeine, and certain foods. Ashley, in our opening story, was experiencing a combination of tension-type and migraine headaches.

TABLE 25.1. COMMON TYPES OF CHRONIC HEADACHE AFTER BRAIN INJURY

Type	Characteristics
Tension-Type	Bilateral, dull pressure-like pain
	Often triggered by stress
Migraine	Often one-sided
	Throbbing pain
	May be associated with nausea, vomiting, or auras (for example, seeing flashes of light)
Occipital Neuralgia	Pain in the back of the head or on top of the head, in the neck, and behind the eyes; tends to be piercing pain
	Pain worsens on neck movement
	Associated with increased sensitivity to light
Cervicogenic	Associated with neck pain and neck stiffness
	May be one-sided or appear on both sides
	Pain worsens in certain neck positions
Medication Overuse	Use of analgesics (ibuprofen, for example, for more than 15 days a month for more than three months)
Other Causes	Bleeding in the brain (sometimes indicated by a very severe headache, the worst in someone's life). *Bleeding in the brain is a medical emergency.* If you suspect there is bleeding in the brain, call 911 immediately!
	Surgery to the brain

Management

There are multiple forms of treatment for headaches following brain injury. For most people, headaches resolve on their own. In cases of chronic headache, medications can help; they are prescribed based on type and cause of the headache. Stress management (with meditation and yoga), talk therapy (particularly cognitive behavioral therapy), exercise, adequate sleep, good nutrition, acupuncture, massage therapy, and support from family and friends are all important factors for alleviating headaches.

Medication

The two approaches to treating migraine headaches are either acute treatment for the current headaches only or regularly taking a medication to prevent or minimize future migraines. Acute treatment usually involves triptan medications such as Imitrex (sumatriptan), Zomig (zolmitriptan), or Relpax (eletriptan). Botox (botulinum toxin) injections can also be helpful for migraines, although Botox is usually reserved for people with chronic migraines.

For people who have frequent migraines, preventive therapy (that is, treatment to prevent or minimize the occurrence of headaches in the future) may also be beneficial. Preventive medications include Topamax (topiramate), Depakote (valproic acid), Inderal (propranolol), Effexor (venlafaxine), and Aimovig (erenumab). Topamax (topiramate) may also help with impulsivity after brain injury. Depakote (valproic acid), a mainstay of bipolar disorder treatment, may also help with irritability and agitation, which may develop after brain injury. Incidentally, both Topamax (topiramate) and Depakote (valproic acid) are antiseizure medications. Inderal (propranolol) is a medication for high blood pressure. Effexor (venlafaxine) is also an antidepressant and can be used for anxiety. Aimovig (erenumab) is a newer FDA-approved medication for the prevention of migraine headaches. It is given as an injection once a month. It acts by blocking a protein known as calcitonin gene-related protein, or CGRP, that is increased during the time the person is experiencing headaches. Other similar approved medications are given as injections: Ajovy (fremanezumab), Emgality (galcanezumab), and Vyepti (eptinezumab), as well as oral agents that block CGRP, such as Nurtec ODT (rimegepant) and Qulipta (atogepant).

There is much overlap in the uses of these medications, so if the person with brain injury is having multiple symptoms or medical problems, their physician may prescribe one medication to help treat several or all of them.

After brain injury, it is also possible to have a mixed type of headache in which there is both a tension-type headache component and a migraine component, as Ashley experienced. These headache combinations can be challenging to treat, especially if they occur frequently months to years after the brain injury. Mood problems like depression can complicate some people's response to medication. Depression and migraines (and possibly other types of headache) may make each other worse. There may also be some overlap in the neurophysiology and neurotransmitters involved. For example, medications that increase serotonin are mainstays of treatment for both depression and migraine (although they are different types of medication). Treatment of depression or anxiety may be a critical part of recovery from chronic headaches.

It is also possible that the headaches after brain injury are not due to the injury at all, or at least not *exclusively* to the brain injury. Headaches are common throughout the general population and are not always the result of a brain injury. The onset of headaches after brain injury, especially chronic headaches, may be a coincidence. It could also be that the life changes and stresses associated with sustaining a brain injury might trigger headaches in someone who was already vulnerable to getting headaches (because of genetics, for example). Sometimes headaches are accompanied by other symptoms, such as vertigo. Treating the vertigo may help, as vertigo can sometimes contribute to headache symptoms. Vertigo is experienced as a sensation of spinning of either the person or the environment around them. Vertigo may be due to an inner ear problem or brain injury itself.

In summary, headaches are not uncommon after brain injury. Often, especially with chronic headaches, there are multiple factors involved. Mood problems, sleep disturbances, stress, and even certain medications can all affect whether someone has headaches after brain injury and what kind of headaches they have.

Tips and tools on how to manage the symptoms discussed in this chapter appear in tables 25.2 and 25.3.

TABLE 25.2. TIPS AND TOOLS FOR COPING WITH HEADACHES AFTER BRAIN INJURY

Get Help	If headaches are severe, chronic, persistent, or associated with vomiting or blurred vision, contact your primary care doctor.
Keep a Healthy Lifestyle	Maintain a healthy lifestyle. Despite the headache, try to get some form of regular exercise.
	Keep a structured daily routine, stay engaged with hobbies, practice good sleep hygiene (see chapter 20).
	Take steps to manage your stress.
Find Your Stress Buster	Find out what relaxes you and do it!
	Meditation techniques such as mindfulness, repeating a mantra (a word or a phrase), or tensing and relaxing parts of your body can help with relaxation.
	Rhythmic breathing or yoga techniques can help as well.
Do Not Overuse Pain Medications	Excessive use of pain medications, such as triptans like Imitrex (sumatriptan) or non-steroidal anti-inflammatory drugs like Motrin (ibuprofen) can make headaches worse.

Table 25.2 continued on next page

| Get Professional Help | If you have mood, anxiety, or other emotional symptoms, consult a psychiatrist or therapist. |
| | These professionals can make appropriate referrals if you need more or different approaches to headache treatment than they have to offer. |

TABLE 25.3. TIPS AND TOOLS FOR CARING FOR SOMEONE WITH HEADACHES AFTER BRAIN INJURY

Offer Reassurance and Support	You can also help by providing the person anything that is comforting: a massage, ice pack, or a cool rag.
The Pain Is Real for the Person	Minimizing it, negating it, or saying "It's only a headache" is not helpful.
Get Professional Help	Encourage the person to get help from a professional with expertise in headaches and brain injury.

The dos and don'ts of caring for headaches, as discussed in this chapter, appear in table 25.4.

TABLE 25.4. DOS AND DON'TS FOR HEADACHE MANAGEMENT

Dos	Don'ts
Maintain a healthy lifestyle: regular exercise and a healthy diet.	Avoid foods that trigger headaches and excessive use of pain meds.
Caregiver: Show that you care that they are in pain and that you are there for them.	*Caregiver:* Don't pressure the person to follow a schedule or be involved in an activity when they are in pain. If the person wants to be alone, give them space.

Caregiver: Think outside the box. Be creative and think about other strategies that may help, but do consult with the person's health care professional before enforcing.

Caregiver: Do not fall into the trap of making pain the person's identity. Help the person juggle the balance between pain and life.

Take-Home Points

Headaches are not unusual after brain injury.

There are multiple factors associated with headache after brain injury. Depression, anxiety, post-traumatic stress disorder, and sleep problems are often co-occurring problems, and when untreated, they tend to worsen headaches.

Treatment includes managing the acute symptoms if severe with medications and managing the chronic symptoms with a combination of medications that have potential to prevent headaches and therapies to reduce stress and improve relaxation.

Start by connecting with your primary care clinician.

Exercise

Manage **PAIN**

• **P**rescription medications. Use medicines and doses prescribed by your doctor to treat acute headaches, prevent headaches, and treat other emotional and physical health problems.

• **A**ctivities. Keep up with daily exercise, leisure, and relaxation activities.

• **I**dentify and pursue triggers for your headaches.

• **N**o—Say no to alcohol, excess caffeine, tobacco, foods that trigger headaches, and excessive pain meds.

Chapter 26

Seizures

Rashad, a 33-year-old architect, sustained a severe traumatic brain injury when three men assaulted him in the alley behind his office. The men surrounded Rashad and demanded his wallet. When he refused, they beat him, kicked him repeatedly in the head and neck, then robbed him and left him sprawled in the alley. A passerby, who found him bleeding from his nose, with fluid draining from his ears, called 911 for help. An ambulance rushed Rashad to the emergency department. By this time, Rashad was unresponsive. Examination showed he had multiple contusions and bleeding inside his brain. Rashad was admitted to the neurocritical care unit and underwent brain surgery to remove a blood clot. He received antiseizure medication for seven days. After two weeks in the neurocritical care unit, he was transferred to an inpatient rehabilitation facility, where he continued to make good progress. He was discharged five weeks after the assault.

Rashad continued to do well after returning home, but about six months after the injury he began to have seizures. His seizures would start with jerking movements of his right hand and soon be followed by jerking movements of all four of his extremities, along with loss of consciousness. Sometimes he would cry out or scream aloud as he lost consciousness and fell to the ground, and sometimes he would lose control of his bladder and urinate. A typical episode would last for a couple of minutes, but he would be confused and groggy for about four to six hours after the event. Rashad would have about three or four such seizures a month. A neurologist evaluated Rashad, diagnosed him with secondarily generalized post-traumatic seizures, as he had no previous history of seizures and no family history of seizures.

Symptoms

Seizures can occur immediately after a traumatic brain injury (within the first 24 hours), early (within the first week), or late (beyond the first week). Late seizures have the highest risk of leading to an ongoing seizure disorder called epilepsy. Seizures are often associated with mood, cognitive, or behavioral problems, and they can complicate recovery from brain injury. Also, the onset of repeated seizures in adulthood without any previous history or without trauma to the head can be suggestive of an acquired brain injury.

What Is a Seizure?

Seizures, or convulsions, happen when the brain's electrical system malfunctions. Normally, the brain discharges electrical energy in an organized, controlled manner that permits the brain cells to communicate with one another. But when the brain's electrical system malfunctions, the brain cells fire in a disorganized manner and keep on firing. The resulting surge of energy through the brain causes a loss of consciousness and muscle contractions.

Seizures can last anywhere from a few seconds to a couple of minutes, but the person often is confused after a seizure, and this post-seizure confusion can last for minutes or as long as several hours. A seizure that persists for several minutes is a medical emergency requiring immediate hospitalization. Epilepsy is a disorder in which a person experiences more than two unprovoked seizures.

Seizures are categorized as partial or generalized. Partial seizures affect only part of the brain. Generalized seizures affect the entire brain. A secondarily generalized seizure is a partial seizure that spreads and becomes generalized. This form of seizure is common after a brain injury. Rashad, in our opening story, developed secondarily generalized seizures.

Generalized Seizures

The classic image of seizure—someone getting stiff and shaking—is in fact a type of generalized seizure called a tonic-clonic seizure, or grand mal seizure. In this kind of seizure, the person loses consciousness and may bite their tongue or lose control of their bladder. They are usually tired and confused after the seizure. Tonic-clonic seizures can be scary to witness, but they are even more dangerous to the person having the seizure. If you see someone having a tonic-clonic seizure, call 911 to bring emergency medical technicians to evaluate the person. A tonic-clonic seizure that lasts more than a few minutes increases the risk of cutting off oxygen to the brain and causing subsequent brain damage.

Partial Seizures

A partial seizure is less obvious than a generalized tonic-clonic seizure. Partial seizures are subdivided into simple partial seizures, in which the person does not lose awareness or become confused, and complex partial seizures, in which the person either loses awareness or becomes confused during the time of the seizure.

The manifestations of a partial seizure vary by the location in the brain. If the seizure is in the frontal lobe, the person can feel that someone or something is forcing thoughts or actions on them. Temporal lobe seizures create a sense of fear, déjà vu (the feeling that one has already seen or experienced something), a rising sensation from the abdomen (like the feeling on a roller coaster), and even hallucinations and the sense that things are not real. Temporal lobe seizures can lead to vertigo or trouble with speech. Parietal lobe seizures can lead to odd body sensations. Occipital lobe seizures can lead to visual hallucinations. As you can see, partial seizures can be difficult to recognize.

A person having a partial seizure can experience mood changes (sadness, anger, fear), cognitive changes (feeling as if they are in a dream, mystical experiences, memory problems), or psychotic symptoms (such as hallucinations) before, during, or after the seizure.

If any one of these changes occurs at the time of the seizure, it can be hard to determine whether the symptoms indicate a seizure. A key factor to consider is how long the symptoms last. Seizures can last from a few seconds to a few minutes. Another factor is that seizures are stereotyped to each person, which means that the symptoms appear essentially the same in that person for each seizure.

Partial seizures can induce a panicky sensation, which can be hard to differentiate from a panic attack. Again, remember that seizures last from seconds to minutes, whereas panic attacks tend to last longer. Seizures occur suddenly, often without warning. Panic attacks may build up over time and can be brought on by a stressor or trigger (such as being in enclosed spaces for those who have claustrophobia). The panic or fear from a seizure, on the other hand, does not build up; it occurs at a maximum level immediately.

Seizures can cause other anxiety symptoms that are easily confused with anxiety disorders. A person having a seizure may feel that the world around him is not real (derealization) or that he himself is not real (depersonalization). Such surreal experiences can lead to anxiety. Partial seizures originating in the temporal lobe can cause these sensations; partial seizures affecting the amygdala (near the temporal lobe) can lead to panic.

Besides panic and anxiety, partial seizures that affect the temporal lobe can lead to cognitive issues like memory impairment, déjà vu, or psychotic symptoms.

Brain injury can also cause complex partial seizure episodes that in some way impair the person's consciousness. The person may be confused or completely unaware of their surroundings during such seizures. Complex partial seizures often can originate in the temporal and frontal lobes, and given that these areas are particularly vulnerable to injury, such seizures may occur after TBI in particular.

Why do some people have seizures after traumatic brain injury and others do not? The answer may lie in part with the severity of the TBI. The more severe the TBI, the more likely it is, in general, that seizures will develop. Bleeding in the brain increases the risk of seizures, partly because blood irritates the brain. Penetrating brain injuries (in which an object penetrates the scalp and brain) are more likely to lead to seizures than are closed-head injuries (in which there is no penetration). Increased age and a family history of epilepsy also increase the risk of developing seizures after a TBI.

Having a seizure within the first 24 hours to a week after the TBI does not mean that the person will necessarily develop epilepsy. These early seizures can be a result of physical and metabolic changes in the brain that occurred soon after the injury. Late seizures can be related to structural changes and scarring in the brain.

Epilepsy

Our discussion thus far has focused on the acute issues related to seizures after brain injury. But the person with brain injury who develops epilepsy faces a different set of challenges. First and foremost, it is important to remember that people with brain injury and seizures following brain injury should avoid alcohol, as that might affect the risk of seizures. People with brain injury who have epilepsy have an increased risk of developing mood and anxiety problems. Depression can be common in epilepsy and may even be a greater influence on quality of life than the type or frequency of the seizures. Luckily, depression with epilepsy responds to typically used antidepressants. Treating the depression not only improves quality of life but may also impact the seizures themselves.

People with brain injury who develop epilepsy may also be vulnerable to psychotic hallucinations or delusions as part of the seizure, right after a seizure, or as an ongoing problem between seizures. Treatment with antipsychotics is necessary for some of these people, particularly when psychotic symptoms continue between seizures. If the psychotic symptoms occur during or after seizures, the best treatment may be antiseizure medications.

Nonepileptic Seizures

Some people with brain injury develop nonepileptic seizures (NES), spells that are not detectable with standard diagnostic tests, such as electroencephalogram (EEG). They are unusual in their presentation in some ways. For example, a person experiencing an NES may thrash around, but their arms and legs are not coordinated together as typically happens in epileptic seizures, or they may be moving all parts of their body but be able to respond at the same time. NES is considered a conversion disorder. We don't understand conversion disorder very well, but we do know that in some people, psychological symptoms "convert" to neurological symptoms such as seizures. Conversion is not malingering; that is, the person who has these symptoms is not knowingly making them up. Rather, we believe subconscious mental stress or distress generates these symptoms. Nonepileptic seizures are best treated by working with a psychiatrist, a psychologist, or a therapist. Treatment of underlying distress along with the *acceptance* by the person with brain injury that their seizure-like symptoms may be from underlying distress can help improve the symptoms.

It can be difficult, however, even for experts to distinguish nonepileptic seizures from epilepsy. To complicate this further, some people with epileptic seizures can also experience NES. Also, an EEG may not detect the source if the seizure originated deep within the brain. EEG electrodes are placed on the scalp, so the seizures they capture best are those near the scalp. The type of EEG may be a factor in picking up a seizure: a regular EEG is not as sensitive in picking up seizures as an ambulatory EEG, which records electrical activity over 24 or 48 hours. Even more effective is monitoring for 48 or 72 hours in an inpatient epilepsy monitoring unit. Even under these conditions, it is possible to miss a deep seizure, though if there was a seizure with no EEG correlation, that is typically suggestive of an NES. Finally, a seizure disorder cannot always be ruled out even if the patient shows no clinical symptoms (and hence no EEG abnormalities) during monitoring.

Management

People who have early seizures after an acute brain injury such as a traumatic brain injury are often treated with antiseizure medications for about a week to prevent further seizures and brain damage from lack of oxygen. Even those who have not had seizures but appear to be at risk are treated with antiseizure medications for about a week. Rashad did not have an early seizure, but because he had a severe injury, his doctors considered him to be at risk and prescribed antiseizure medication for the first week after injury. In situations where a brain tumor or hemorrhagic stroke is causing seizures, treatment of the brain tumor or stroke may eliminate ongoing seizures, though not always, and people are often prescribed antiseizure medications for at least some period of time.

People who have late-onset seizures receive medication after the seizures begin. The neurologist determines when to start and stop antiseizure medications and what type of medicine to use. The onset of late seizures is unpredictable; evidence shows an elevated risk for a first seizure 10 or even 20 years after severe brain injury (particularly TBI).

Antiepileptic medications can have mood, behavioral, and cognitive side effects. Certain antiepileptics, like Topamax (topiramate) and Dilantin (phenytoin), can cause cognitive side effects (problems with memory or finding the right word when needed). Keppra (levetiracetam) can lead to irritability, agitation, and depression in some patients. On the other hand, if the person with brain injury has trouble with mood stability, some antiepileptic medications, such as Lamictal (lamotrigine), Depakote (valproic acid), or Tegretol (carbamazepine), may be helpful with mood as well as seizure control. Lyrica (pregabalin) or Neurontin (gabapentin) may help the person with brain injury who has anxiety problems. Another thing to be aware of is the potential for unintended interactions between antiepileptics and other medications the person with brain injury is taking, because such interactions can affect both the person's tolerance and the effectiveness of the antiepileptic. Therefore, it is extremely important that a neuropsychiatrist or neurologist trained in brain injury be managing medications.

In summary, seizures can occur after brain injury and are more common in moderate and severe brain injury than in mild injury. Seizures can manifest in many different ways: they can be partial or generalized or start partially and become generalized. In addition, seizures can occur with or without loss of consciousness. Emotional and behavioral problems are common in people with seizures.

If you or the person you are caring for has had seizures after brain injury, seek professional help from a neurologist and follow their recommendations. Having a seizure or seizures after brain injury is no guarantee that epilepsy (that is, recurrent seizures) will develop. On the other hand, there can be an increased risk of seizures years after the brain injury. The good news is that there are a number of medications to treat seizures, and chances are good that these medications will control the seizures.

Tips and tools on how to manage the symptoms discussed in this chapter appear in tables 26.1 and 26.2.

TABLE 26.1. TIPS AND TOOLS FOR COPING WITH SEIZURES AFTER BRAIN INJURY	
Educate Yourself	Educate yourself by reading and talking to your health care professionals about brain injury and seizures.
Avoid Alcohol and Street Drugs	This is a must! Alcohol, certain street drugs, excess caffeine, and energy drinks can lower your threshold for having seizures and put you at risk for both more frequent and longer-lasting seizures—both of which are bad for your brain.

Table 26.1 continued on next page

Get a Medical Alert Necklace or Bracelet	This can help other people observing a seizure get you medical help immediately.
	Sometimes the seizure activity or confusion following a seizure can be misperceived as inappropriate behavior by people, and police may be called. Having the medical alert identifier will be beneficial in getting the medical help you need.

TABLE 26.2. TIPS AND TOOLS FOR CARING FOR SOMEONE WITH SEIZURES AFTER BRAIN INJURY

Emphasize Safety	Safety comes first and trumps all other issues.
	Keep the person having a seizure safe.
	If they are seated and having a seizure, hold them to make sure they do not fall over.
	If they are standing, gently lower them to the floor.
	Turn them onto their left side to prevent them from aspirating saliva into the lungs.
	Loosen any tight clothes around their neck.
	Do not put anything in their mouth.
	Do not try to restrain the person.
Call 911	Call 911 if
	• this is the first time the person is having a seizure,
	• the seizure lasts longer than three minutes, or
	• the person does not wake up after 15 minutes.
	If the person has had seizures before or if the seizure lasts less than three minutes, do not call 911 but do inform their doctor of the episode.
Be a Partner	Use the buddy system for high-risk activities.
	People who have post–brain injury seizures should never be alone when performing activities such as bathing, swimming, climbing heights, or operating machinery.

Educate Yourself	Learn your state's regulations on driving.
	A person with post–brain injury seizures should consult their neurologist and follow their recommendations about when it is safe to drive again. States' regulations vary regarding how long someone must be seizure-free before they are allowed to drive.
Be on the Watch for Other Problems	If you notice mood, cognitive, or behavioral symptoms in the person with brain injury and seizures, encourage them to consult their doctor.
	They may need additional treatment from a psychiatrist or a therapist.
Know Their Triggers	Be alert to specific triggers that provoke seizures.
	Common triggers include bright lights, alcohol or illicit drug use, alcohol withdrawal, and irregular sleep patterns.
	For people who are prescribed antiseizure medication, the most common trigger for a seizure is not taking the medication.

Take-Home Points

Seizures can occur immediately after a brain injury, particularly a TBI (within the first 24 hours), early (within the first week), or late (beyond the first week).

Seizures are often associated with mood, cognitive, or behavioral problems, and they can complicate recovery from brain injury.

Consultation with your doctors and compliance with treatment will greatly help in controlling the seizures and other associated symptoms.

Exercise
Think **ABC** to prevent seizures

• **A**void alcohol, energy drinks, excess caffeine.

• **B**etter lifestyle. Work with your health care professionals to better your lifestyle with strategies to reduce stress, minimize fatigue, and improve sleep.

• **C**ompliance with medications and treatment.

Chapter 27

Vision

Staff Sergeant Patrice's third tour of duty in Afghanistan ended with an explosion. She and her unit hit an improvised explosive device as they rode cautiously through a deserted town. The explosion slammed Patrice, who was riding inside the tank, up against the roof. She and the other surviving soldiers radioed for help and were airlifted back to base, where medical personnel diagnosed Patrice with a broken left arm and a moderate traumatic brain injury. Within two days, 30-year-old Patrice was recovering at an army medical center back in the United States.

Although Patrice's arm healed quickly, her brain injury led to several physical problems, including difficulties with walking, balance, speech, and vision. Her visual problems included increased sensitivity to light, blurred vision, and, periodically, double vision. The examining physician noted that Patrice had difficulty moving her eyes in all directions. These visual problems were very troubling to Patrice, and she wondered if she would ever be able to do what she could do before. "I'm seeing double so much of the time now," she said. "I'm always knocking my coffee cup over."

Traumatic brain injury can lead to a range of vision problems, including double vision, trouble keeping the eyes in place while reading (maintaining focus), blurred vision, sensitivity to light, eye strain, depth perception dysfunction, and inability to see part of the environment. Chronic visual problems are more common in moderate to severe TBI than in mild TBI, though people can have problems with their vision (like double or blurry vision) for a few days to weeks after a mild TBI. Diagnosing and treating visual problems in TBI is particularly important because any visual disturbance, no matter how slight, can impact a person's life, including their rehabilitation, impeding their ability to fully participate in and improve with physical therapy after TBI. Furthermore, because vision is a critical sense for us, sudden and traumatically induced visual problems can be very disconcerting to people, and they can contribute to depression and anxiety problems.

The specific visual problem that occurs depends on the location of the brain damage and the severity of the injury. Visual problems can originate in any of the multiple regions in the brain that transmit and process visual information. Damage to the eye itself or the optic nerve (which connects the eyes to the brain) can also result in the onset of vision difficulties after a brain injury.

How Brain Injury Affects Vision

Brain injury can directly damage the eyes and the optic nerves. In a car accident, for example, the impact can propel the driver through the windshield, directly traumatizing the face and eyes. People with damage to the retina, the layer of cells in the back of the eyeball, may see floaters (or floating spots), small pieces of tissue floating within the eyeball. Direct or indirect injury to the optic nerves (called traumatic optic neuropathy) is one of the most serious visual problems that can result from TBI.

Brain injury can damage the visual pathways connecting the cell groupings in the brain that process visual information. Because each of these cell groupings carries out different functions, damage to them leads to different visual symptoms.

When we look out at the world, we usually assume that our brain is faithfully reproducing the world out there. In truth, however, what we see is an illusion. Instead, the brain builds a model of visual reality out of information that it receives through the eyes. The world "out there" is composed of light that oscillates at different frequencies, some of which we can see and some of which we cannot (ultraviolet and infrared light are two examples). The brain quickly, efficiently, and automatically converts these light waves into a model of the world that we recognize and assume is there.

This concept may seem radical, but the science leaves no doubt that the brain alone is the architect of the world we see. To illustrate this, consider that our eyes continuously move slightly, even when we are still. Our eyes are moving as we walk, too. But as we walk, we don't see the world as blurred moving images. Instead, we see a stable backdrop because the brain is continually making adjustments to how it perceives the world. Furthermore, even though our eyes project information from the world to our brain upside down our brain inverts the image, so we don't even know that the information we had originally was upside down.

At a deeper level, different parts of the brain receive information describing the color, shape, and movement of an object. The brain has to blend or bind all this information together so that when we look out at the world, we see all aspects of the object simultaneously—that is, we see the color, shape, and other attributes of the object instantly and at the same location in space. The brain combines this information and other information instantaneously, so we don't even know that it is happening or appreciate the amount of work that goes into it.

Brain injury can disrupt the extensive circuitry that carries out these amazing feats. Vision circuitry involves pathways that lead from the retinas to an area called the optic chiasm, and then to the lateral geniculate nucleus of the thalamus. This region of the thalamus combines visual input with other sensory input. The thalamus relays visual information to the occipital cortex (the primary visual center) and to the superior colliculus, in the midbrain, which directs eye movements.

Axons (nerve cell fibers) in the retina at the back of the eye exit the retina bundled together as the optic nerve. At the optic chiasm, a partial joining of information from the two eyes joins the fibers from each eye that receive input from the same place in space. Information reaches the lateral geniculate nucleus of the thalamus on each side and is then relayed to the occipital lobe of each hemisphere of the brain. The left occipital cortex receives information about the right side of the world from both eyes, and the right occipital cortex receives information about the left side of the world from both eyes.

From the occipital cortex, information can travel via either the ventral pathway (the "what" pathway) or the dorsal pathway (the "where" pathway). The ventral pathway passes through the inferior temporal lobe and is associated with recognizing objects ("what" things are). The dorsal pathway passes through the middle temporal lobe to the parietal lobe and is associated with motion and spatial vision ("where" things are).

Where in these circuits the damage occurred determines what specific visual problem a person with brain injury has. Damage to the optic nerve from one eye can lead to complete visual loss from that eye. Damage at the optic chiasm can lead to lack of vision from parts of both eyes. People can also have "holes" in their vision (called scotomas), spots in the visual field where vision is absent or deficient.

A severe traumatic brain injury can impact the fibers that run from the optic chiasm to the thalamus and then to the occipital lobe, causing blindness in part of the visual field from both eyes (called visual field cuts), or scotomas. Damage to the fibers on the right side of the brain can lead to loss of vision on the left visual field and vice versa. Damage to the occipital lobes can lead to total blindness (for example, with a stroke). In a condition called Anton's syndrome, people with damage to the occipital lobes are not able to see, but do not accept that they are blind and confabulate a visual image. Their brains are unable to recognize that they are blind. Although it is challenging to appreciate that a person is experiencing such profound unawareness, the individual is not faking and truly has no awareness of the impairment.

In addition to the fibers connecting the eyes to the occipital lobes are fibers that connect the eyes to specific regions of the brainstem. These areas control eye movements, so damage to these regions can lead to blurry or double vision, the very problems that Patrice complained of in our opening story. Although this condition is more common in cases of moderate and severe TBI, it is not uncommon initially after a mild TBI.

Of the twelve cranial nerves, numbers III, IV, and VI, located in the middle of the brainstem, control the eye movements and can be damaged by injury to the back of the brain, where the brainstem is. Damage to these pathways can impair the ability of both eyes to focus on the same spot, leading to eye strain and blurry vision, or cause uncoordinated movements of the eyes, creating double vision. Severe TBI can misalign one or both eyes. Comprehensive eye examination revealed that Patrice had damage to the nerves responsible for moving the eyes.

Rarely, visual problems can develop from impaired perception of one's surroundings, due to damage to the dorsal visual pathway that leads to the parietal lobe. People who suffer this injury completely neglect one side of space and are aware of and act in only the other side. A man would shave only one side of his face, for example, or a woman would apply makeup to only one eye or put clothes on only one side of her body, simply because they are not aware of the other side of space. This phenomenon (called unilateral spatial neglect) can occur after stroke, particularly a right parietal lobe stroke.

Light sensitivity can also develop after brain injury. The person with TBI may feel pain or discomfort in their eyes when they are exposed to light. We're not sure why this occurs, although one hypothesis is that it is associated with changes in blood flow in the brain after brain injury.

Management

The mainstay of treatment for visual problems after brain injury is visual rehabilitation, a process of educating and training people with visual deficits to achieve maximum visual function and optimal quality of life. Eye doctors (ophthalmologists), optometrists, or a team of specially trained professionals can provide visual rehabilitation. A visual therapist tailors the specific rehabilitation strategy to the source of the problem— the eyes, the optic nerves, the visual areas of the brain, or the cranial nerves in the brainstem. Depression or anxiety symptoms after visual problems should be treated aggressively by the appropriate clinician.

Surgery may be necessary if the retina is damaged or detached from the tissue around it. If the person with brain injury experiences blurred vision and the problem appears to originate in the eyes themselves, then prescription eyeglasses or contact lenses may be appropriate. Refractive prisms may be used in rehabilitation to help the blurriness improve.

If there is damage to the optic nerve, steroids may be used soon after the brain damage; surgery may also be necessary in the early stages of injury. Damage to the visual pathways may require either surgery to remove blood from the brain, or a temporary course of steroids. Unfortunately, moderate and severe brain injury can lead to permanent visual problems because the damage may be subtle or may not be responsive to medical or surgical treatment. In these cases, visual rehabilitation can teach strategies that compensate for lost or diminished vision. Special tinted lenses that decrease light sensitivity, or prism lenses or eye patches to treat double vision, may be helpful.

Because vision is a critical sense to most people, visual problems can lead to anxiety and depressive symptoms. It is important to address these symptoms and treat them, as one's mood can affect rehabilitation and make recovery more difficult. This can become a circular problem, as poor rehabilitation participation can lead to no improvement of symptoms, which can lead to worsening anxiety or depression.

In summary, visual problems can occur after brain injury. Because vision is one of the critical senses and because we rely heavily on visual information to navigate the world, restoring vision quickly is a priority in people with brain injury. Addressing vision problems as quickly as possible after the brain injury maximizes the person's benefit from overall rehabilitation because they are better able to engage in treatment. It is important to address anxiety and depression quickly and aggressively as well.

Tips and tools on how to manage the symptoms discussed in this chapter appear in tables 27.1 and 27.2.

TABLE 27.1. TIPS AND TOOLS FOR COPING WITH VISUAL PROBLEMS AFTER BRAIN INJURY

Go to an Expert	Consult an eye specialist (ophthalmologist or optometrist) if you are concerned about your vision.
	An eye specialist may refer you to a neuro-ophthalmologist (a super-specialist with expertise in brain injury) or to a visual rehabilitation therapist or to both.
Take It Easy	If in addition to visual problems, you are having other issues such as imbalance, headache, or fatigue, try to take it easy. Break down tasks into simple steps and focus on one step at a time.
	Consult with your doctor or vision therapist if you need to see another professional for associated problems such as dizziness, imbalance, headache.
Get Help	Don't be shy about reaching out to family and friends for help.
	You might benefit from someone coming to your home and organizing things for you or someone helping you with day-to-day activities such as cooking, shopping, and other tasks.
	Consider asking your doctor about having a service animal.

TABLE 27.2. TIPS AND TOOLS FOR CARING FOR SOMEONE WITH VISION PROBLEMS AFTER BRAIN INJURY

Organize the Home	Reduce clutter and keep the home organized.
	Simple and powerful tools to help the person with brain injury and visual problems include having clear walking pathways, organized workspaces, and cueing systems to help them identify objects or locations (such as a guide string leading from the kitchen table to the bathroom).

Table 27.1 continued on next page

Provide Support	Offer emotional support.
	Having visual problems after a brain injury can be a very frightening experience.
Think outside the Box	Vision problems can be associated with other physical and emotional problems such as headache, dizziness, anxiety, and depression. If these symptoms are persistent, impacting daily life, or interfering with the ability of your loved one to continue visual therapy, encourage them to seek help with other professionals knowledgeable in brain injury.

Take-Home Points

Brain injury can lead to a range of vision problems such as blurred vision, double vision, sensitivity to light, maintaining eye focus, loss of field vision, or difficulty with depth perception.

Diagnosing and treating visual problems is important as even mild problems can cause significant distress and reduced quality of life.

The type of visual problem depends on the location of the brain injury. Visual problems can originate in the eye, in the nerve that transfers visual information from the eye to the brain (the optic nerve), or in any of the pathways or brain regions that transmit and process visual information.

Visual rehabilitation is the mainstay of treatment. If you have any type of eye problems, consult with your eye doctor, who will be able to make appropriate referrals.

Exercise

Think **VISION**

• **V**ision therapy: consult an eye doctor if you have any type of vision problems.

• **I**mprove eye hygiene: clean your eyes/glasses/contacts; stop smoking, eat healthy (especially yellow and orange-colored vegetables/fruits and leafy vegetables).

• **S**tress reduction helps: be gentle to your eyes and take frequent breaks from any activities that stress your eyes, such as reading, watching TV, or working on a computer, phone, or tablet.

• **I**ncrease font size of reading material; increase contrast between objects and background so that they stand out and are more easily seen.

• **O**rganize your home or workspace to reduce clutter and avoid visual overload.

• **N**eutralize bright lights (like fluorescent lights, strobe flashing lights, and other visually stimulating objects) by removing them or toning them down.

Chapter 28

Balance

Tom was driving on the highway when the car in front of him suddenly braked. He was going around 60 miles an hour, and he could not stop before hitting the car in front of him. The impact of the crash accelerated his head forward, but his airbags deployed, stopping his head from hitting the windshield. After the crash, he experienced headaches, disorientation, and dizziness, and felt off-balance. Over the next few weeks, the headaches and disorientation went away, but the dizziness and unsteadiness continued. He had difficulty getting out of bed and moving without getting dizzy. These symptoms impacted his day-to-day functioning, because he was not able to drive and get to work. He eventually worked with a physical therapist, and over the span of several months, he was able to get better control over his dizziness as well as attaining improved balance and steadiness in his walking.

Symptoms

Let's start by distinguishing between dizziness and vertigo. Dizziness is often used as an umbrella term to describe lightheadedness, faintness, unsteadiness, feeling off-balance, or a spinning sensation. But strictly speaking, dizziness is a sensation of spatial disorientation—a state of confusion of where we are in space and feeling off-balance. Vertigo, on the other hand, is a feeling that your body is spinning or the world around you is spinning.

In this chapter, we focus on balance, as both dizziness and vertigo can lead to a disturbance in balance. For simplicity we use the term *dizziness*, as used by Tom in our story.

Balance is very important in our interaction with the world. Because balance is so automatic, we may not truly appreciate it until there is something that causes dysfunction or imbalance. Brain injuries can cause damage to our balance system. With mild traumatic brain injuries (concussions), for example, balance problems like dizziness can be one of the most bothersome symptoms and often related to an inner ear problem. Other injuries to the brain such as tumors or strokes can also affect our balance system, causing dizziness.

Normal balance is created by multiple systems, the inner ear being one that is critical for our sense of balance. Two organs in the inner ear maintain balance: semicircular canals that mediate rotational or rolling movements (also known as rotational acceleration) and the utricle and saccule, which react to up/down and side-to-side positional changes (also known as linear movements or linear acceleration). As we move our heads, fluids in the semicircular canals and crystals in the utricle and saccule move as well, causing inner ear hair cells to bend and causing sensory receptors to send information about our head position in space to the brain. Traumatic brain injuries often involve acceleration or deceleration of the head in space (such as being in a car crash with the head accelerating into the windshield and decelerating suddenly when hitting the windshield), affecting the semicircular canals and the utricle in the inner ear and input that is sent to the brain, leading to dizziness.

Besides the inner ear, the vestibular system in the brainstem is critical for balance. The vestibular system consists of neurons that get information from the inner ear and create an initial representation of space around the head (and the rest of the body). That is, this system creates a model of where the body is in space with respect to the gravitational field that is all around us. It is important for our brains to know where the body is with respect to gravity so that we know what is up and what is down; down is where there is a greater concentration of gravity, while up is where there is a lesser concentration of gravity. The vestibular system also sends information to the eye muscles, allowing our eyes to remain steady even when our heads are moving; this also allows our eyes to move to a target or track movements. Damage to the brainstem can affect the vestibular system, leading to dizziness. Nystagmus (rapid uncontrollable movements of the eyes) can also occur, a condition in which the eyes are not stationary or moving in a controlled manner, but rather are rapidly moving back and forth.

The vestibular system interacts with the cerebellum, which is also in the back of the brain. The cerebellum is important for a number of important functions, including coordinating our movements so that they are fluid. Damage to the cerebellum can cause difficulty in coordinating movements, as can be seen with alcohol intoxication. The cerebellum uses information from the vestibular system to help with coordination, posture, and balance. Damage to the cerebellum can lead to a sense of dizziness and difficulty navigating through space.

Another important system for balance is our proprioceptive system. Proprioception is often coupled with our sense of touch. Proprioception encodes where our limbs (in particular) are in space. It is important for the brain to know where the limbs are in order to program our limbs to move appropriately to avoid obstacles or to grab items. Proprioception information is transmitted to the spinal cord along with touch information, eventually going to the parietal lobe. The parietal lobe is important in ultimately taking all this information and making representations or models of space around our body.

Finally, it is also important to consider mood reasons for dizziness and imbalance, especially anxiety. There is actually a reciprocal relationship between dizziness/imbalance and anxiety. In some people, extreme anxiety can cause dizziness and imbalance, and in some, dizziness/imbalance can cause anxiety. Also, in some people who have panic attacks and breathe rapidly, dizziness can follow the attacks, as the rapid breathing can be associated with decreased carbon dioxide in the body, triggering a sensation of dizziness. A careful evaluation by your doctor can help.

Damage to a number of systems can lead to balance problems. Because multiple systems are involved, multiple types of medical specialists may be needed to make a proper assessment. These specialists can be from neurology, ENT (ear, nose, and throat), neuro-ophthalmology, physical medicine and rehabilitation, psychiatry, and psychology. Diagnostic tests that may be done include brain imaging (typically an MRI), audiologic or hearing testing, and ENG/VNG tests (electro- or videonystagmography). ENG/VNG involves producing and analyzing eye movements electrically or by video recording. Ultimately, diagnostic testing may help to localize the balance problem to either the inner ear or the brain, and then if the problem is in the brain, whether it is due more to vestibular, cerebellar, or proprioceptive system damage.

Management

The management of balance problems depends on where the problem lies. Taking a careful history and doing a comprehensive evaluation by a clinician with expertise in this area will help to determine the cause and presence or absence of other potential associated symptoms (such as ringing in the ears, hearing loss, nausea, vomiting, or decreased sensation in limbs).

For example, if the problem is in the inner ear, there are exercises involving moving the inner ear/head in certain ways (Epley Maneuver; see box) to help improve dizziness. Even though this can be done at home, we suggest that you first practice with your therapist before practicing by yourself at home. Your partner or family member can also learn the steps from your therapist and work with you.

Vestibular therapy can also help with dizziness, be it related to the inner ear or the brain. Vestibular therapy is a physical and occupational therapy procedure that involves exercises with head movements. The idea is to retrain brain systems to assess orientation in space properly. It is made up of a number of elements, including exercises to help the brain overcome dysfunctional responses to head movements after the injury. Postural control exercises are also part of vestibular therapy, helping the brain relearn how to keep a proper upright posture.

Vision therapy may also be appropriate if there is any kind of vision

Epley Maneuver

Follow these steps if the problem is with your right ear:

- Start by sitting on a bed.
- Turn your head 45 degrees to the right.
- Quickly lie back, keeping your head turned. Your shoulders should now be on the pillow, and your head should be reclined. Wait 30 seconds.
- Turn your head 90 degrees to the left, without raising it. Your head will now be looking 45 degrees to the left. Wait another 30 seconds.
- Turn your head and body another 90 degrees to the left, into the bed. Wait another 30 seconds.
- Sit up on the left side.

If the problem is in your left ear, the same steps apply but with your head turned in the opposite direction.

impairment. A reaction or reflex known as the vestibulo-ocular reflex (VOR) is important in stabilizing gaze and balance. The VOR responds immediately to head movements by bringing about eye movements in the direction opposite to the head movements. In other words, the VOR coordinates head and eye movements to maintain steady vision and balance. TBI can cause disruption of the VOR, leading to dizziness, imbalance, or blurred vision. There are many types of visual therapies to coordinate eye movements and balance. Your visual therapist will be able to determine the most appropriate therapy after a careful evaluation.

Overall conditioning exercises are also often done to help the body overcome deconditioning or weakness after injury. There are a variety of conditioning exercises to help improve your physical strength, mobility, and balance, all of which can also improve your coordination, emotional health, and cognitive functions. Your physical therapist will be able to recommend the most appropriate conditioning exercise for you.

Sometimes, your doctor may prescribe other medications to treat associated symptoms such as nausea or vomiting. Or sometimes your doctor may have to reduce the dosage or discontinue certain medications that may be contributing to the balance problem (as certain medications can contribute to balance issues).

In summary, maintaining proper balance involves multiple brain systems. Brain injury of any of these systems can lead to a sense of dizziness, which can be very impairing. Addressing the underlying dysfunction as well as rehabilitation exercises can help over time.

Tips and tools on how to manage the symptoms discussed in this chapter appear in tables 28.1 and 28.2.

TABLE 28.1. TIPS AND TOOLS FOR COPING WITH BALANCE PROBLEMS AFTER BRAIN INJURY

Consult with a Professional	Consultation and evaluation by a health care professional with expertise in the area is a must.
Follow the Treatment Plan	Strictly follow the treatment plan prepared by your therapist.
	Either underdoing or overdoing recommended exercises can hurt.
Exercise Caution	Sit up slowly from a lying position.
	Hold on to something as you stand up from a sitting/lying position. Wait for a minute or so before you start walking.
	Stop and quickly find a safe place to rest if you feel dizzy during any of your activities.

Table 28.1 continued on next page

Maintain a Healthy Lifestyle	It is important to take care of yourself and maintain nutrition and hydration.
	Take medications as prescribed and consult your doctor regarding side effects.
	Avoid alcohol and street drugs as they can also affect your balance.
	Follow good sleep habits.

TABLE 28.2. TIPS AND TOOLS FOR CARING FOR SOMEONE WITH BALANCE PROBLEMS AFTER BRAIN INJURY

Buddy Up	Your loved one may find it difficult or boring to follow or keep up with the exercise plan.
	If you can just be there with them as they practice, or even do some of the exercises with them, it can be very helpful and even fun.
Be Involved	Because there are many reasons for imbalance after brain injury, make sure that other aspects of brain injury are being taken care of by helping the person get regular medical checkups and other treatments deemed necessary.

TAKE-HOME POINTS

Normal balance is maintained by multiple systems and therefore, many things can impact balance.

Comprehensive evaluation by a clinician with expertise in the field of brain injury and balance can help determine the cause and appropriate treatment.

Exercise

• *Know your triggers.*

• *With the help of your therapist, work on an exercise plan that you can do to gradually minimize symptoms that trigger your balance problem.*

• *For example, if the balance problem is related to dizziness, identify activities that trigger dizziness. If moving your head quickly triggers dizziness and imbalance, work on a head-movement exercise plan with your therapist that gently reduces dizziness and improves balance.*

Chapter 29

Hormonal Abnormalities

B ill is a 43-year-old male who had a childhood-onset brain tumor that affected his pituitary gland. He was diagnosed at a young age because the tumor had started to affect his optic tract near the pituitary, which had affected his vision. He had to have radiation treatment to control the tumor growth, but that led to further damage to the pituitary. He started to have difficulty regulating his moods and started getting uncharacteristically irritable. His irritability became a big enough problem over the years that it significantly affected his relationships with his family. He started hormone replacement therapy, and over time, his mood improved, and he experienced only occasional irritability.

Brain injuries can affect hormone levels in the body, which can cause a number of mood, behavioral, and cognitive consequences. Damage to the brain by direct trauma (such as in a traumatic brain injury) or by a brain tumor (such as with Bill) or by other means, such as stroke, can be associated with hormonal imbalances.

The hypothalamus, deep within the brain, causes secretion of hormones from the pituitary gland, which in turn affects organs outside of the brain (such as the adrenal glands above the kidneys) or the thyroid gland. Hormones that can be affected by hypothalamus or pituitary gland injury include glucocorticoids (also known as stress hormones), thyroid hormones, prolactin, oxytocin, antidiuretic hormone, growth hormone, and reproductive hormones.

Abnormalities in glucocorticoid levels (particularly cortisol) can significantly impact mood, behavior, and cognition. Cortisol is secreted by the adrenal glands after stimulation by the hypothalamus and pituitary gland. Cortisol is important in the acute stress response—if someone is chasing after you with a knife, you want to have your body ready to fight or flee. Cortisol allows your body to do this by increasing blood sugar and blood pressure (to have energy), among other things.

With chronic stress and brain injury, however, these responses to cortisol are not helpful. Chronic cortisol release with chronic stress can negatively affect your blood sugar and blood pressure, and cortisol can also impair memory as it can reduce the size of the hippocampus (which is important for short-term memory and conversion to long-term memory), though the stress associated with clinical depression and post-traumatic stress disorder can be potential contributory factors for hippocampal size reduction as well.

The hippocampus acts as a check to cortisol release, and cortisol in turn decreases the effectiveness of the hippocampus. Over time, with chronic release of cortisol, the hippocampus is less and less able to affect additional cortisol release, leading potentially to a runaway cycle, with the stress response gone amok. This, in turn, can lead to the development of mood (depressive) and anxiety disorders.

Thyroid abnormalities can also occur with hypothalamic or pituitary injury. Thyroid hormones are important for optimizing metabolism in nearly every organ system in the body. Low thyroid hormones (hypothyroidism) can be associated with physical symptoms such as fatigue, weight gain, trouble tolerating cold temperatures, and dry skin. Hypothyroidism can also cause neuropsychiatric symptoms such as depression and poor memory. With decreased thyroid hormone activity, the brain can have a significant global decrease in activity, leading to these neuropsychiatric symptoms.

Reproductive hormone levels can also be affected by injuries to the hypothalamus or pituitary. Surprisingly, perhaps, abnormalities in these hormones can also cause neuropsychiatric symptoms. Progesterone, for example, may affect the neurotransmitter gamma aminobutyric acid (GABA) in the brain; GABA is the major inhibitory neurotransmitter in the brain (meaning that it is important in tamping down on neuron firing). If there is a deficiency of progesterone due to brain injury, there can be excess brain activity, which can be manifested with symptoms such as anxiety and irritability. A deficiency in testosterone, on the other hand, can lead to less dominance and aggression.

Oxytocin and antidiuretic hormone (also known as vasopressin) can affect social cognition. Oxytocin may be important in terms of social attachment, especially between mother and child. Decreased oxytocin can lead to decreased trust and attachment. Decreased antidiuretic hormone can lead to decreased aggression, but also decreased social attachment.

Although hormonal abnormalities are not always considered after a brain injury, it is important to keep in mind how brain injuries can in fact cause hormonal disruptions. These disruptions, in turn, can cause significant neuropsychiatric symptoms, ranging from depression to memory problems to decreased social functioning. The good news is there is hope and treatment for hormonal abnormalities, as hormone replacement therapy is generally available to treat these deficiencies.

A neuroendocrinologist has expertise in evaluating and treating hormonal issues after brain injury. Your doctor will be able to make a referral to this specialist. If you are concerned about hormonal issues after brain injury, please talk to your doctor. With early detection and testing, many of the hormonal problems caused by brain injury are treatable.

TAKE-HOME POINTS

Hormonal abnormalities may occur after brain injury.

Untreated hormonal abnormalities can be associated with a variety of emotional, cognitive, and behavioral problems.

Consult with your doctor if you are concerned; your doctor may either be able to do the assessment and provide treatment or refer you to a specialist.

Part VII

The Traumatized Brain *and the* Future

In this last part of the book, we discuss brain injury topics that are still controversial or in the research stage. We discuss what may happen with repeated brain injuries (chapter 30) and, on a more positive note, what future treatments for brain injury may look like (chapter 31).

Repeated
Brain Injuries

Brain injuries are difficult enough to deal with when they occur once. Unfortunately, brain injuries can occur repetitively. There is some controversy in the scientific literature about whether repeated brain injuries can lead to neurodegenerative disease (like dementia). However, most would agree that repeated injuries are clearly not good for the brain, and it is important to try to avoid another brain injury if possible.

It is not uncommon for people to have repeated brain injuries, particularly in the context of mild traumatic brain injuries (concussions). In fact, people can be more vulnerable to having a concussion after they have had their first one. Concussions can occur in sports, for example, and continued playing of the sport can lead to additional concussions. Common symptoms following a concussion make up a long list, including the following: headache; dizziness; imbalance; visual problems; fatigue; increased sensitivity to noise, light, or any kind of stimuli; increased emotionality such as sadness, anxiety, or irritability; and cognitive issues such as fogginess, feeling slowed down, difficulty processing information, difficulty with concentration/attention, short-term memory problems, and difficulty planning, organizing, and executing even simple tasks.

Emergency medical care should be sought if there has been any loss of consciousness and if there are persistent, distressing, or new onset of symptoms such as headaches, seizures, repeated vomiting, blurred vision, or imbalance.

It is important after a first concussion to minimize physical and mental activity immediately afterward to improve symptoms such as headaches, dizziness, or cognitive problems. In general, it is important to rest for one to two days after a concussion. Rest includes both physical and mental rest—no watching television, checking phone messages or texts, or being in crowded places or places where there is loud noise or bright lights. Light activities can be started after about 48 to 72 hours. Depending on the resolution or persistence of symptoms, activities can be gradually upgraded from light to heavy to regular everyday activities.

Of course, it is important to follow your doctor's advice and keep up with the recommendations and treatment plan, because each patient is unique and recovers differently. It is important not to rush recovery or skip treatment. A commonly used adage in the sports world—"when in doubt, sit it out"—can be used by anyone who has had a concussion: if you are experiencing any symptoms following a concussion, get professional help immediately.

Most concussion symptoms do resolve on their own typically over a few weeks. However, some people's symptoms do not resolve even after a year. Many reasons can account for this variation, including multiple concussions, mechanism of injury, extent of white matter damage, older age, presence of either pre-injury or post-injury emotional and medical problems, alcohol and illicit drug use, person's coping style, the stress of ongoing legal issues, and yet other unknown factors.

If a person with a concussion gets a second concussion before the resolution of the first one, symptoms can build on themselves, and rarely can even cause brain swelling and potentially death (this is called second-impact syndrome, or SIS). It is thus important to minimize risk of a second concussion while still recovering from the first one. Minimizing contact sports, for example, is a good idea after a first concussion until resolution of symptoms.

If there are repeated brain injuries over time, it is possible that they can add up and can be followed by long-lasting and/or recurrent emotional, behavioral, physical, and cognitive problems, including dementia. We do know there are cases of boxers who had repeated impacts to the head that developed what is known as dementia pugilistica (colloquially known as punch-drunk syndrome). Dementia can be of various types, but memory problems and behavioral changes can commonly occur. With dementia pugilistica, symptoms can include memory and thinking problems, as well as symptoms seen in Parkinson's disease such as tremor and slowed movements.

There has been recent interest in the media regarding chronic traumatic encephalopathy (CTE); dementia pugilistica may be one example. CTE is a diagnosis made by pathologists after examining the brain after death; currently, there is not a clear way to make the diagnosis in the living brain.

CTE has been linked with repeated concussions. This diagnosis has most commonly been given to professional athletes, such as National Football League (NFL) football players. Oftentimes, the family of the person with repeated brain injuries will have noticed mood, behavioral, and cognitive changes in their loved one. After death (in some cases by suicide), the family may have pathologists examine the brain for CTE. Although a majority of such cases have been diagnosed as having CTE, we do not know how prevalent it actually is in the general population or even among professional football players (as there could be many people who have repeated brain injuries who never develop mood, behavioral, or cognitive symptoms to warrant a pathological examination and diagnosis of CTE).

There is some scientific literature to suggest that CTE may eventually occur after repeated brain injuries due to damage to the axons of neurons in the brain. Damage to axons may lead to a cascade of events, including the abnormal accumulation of a protein called tau. Tau aggregation inside the neuron can lead to what are called neurofibrillary tangles. These abnormally folded and aggregated proteins can lead to death of the neuron and eventually dementia symptoms. However, there is also some scientific literature to suggest that the pathology of CTE is not unique to repetitive trauma. It can be seen even in other neurodegenerative disorders and brain conditions such as amyotrophic lateral sclerosis (ALS). There is thus still a lot we don't know about CTE, and our understanding will hopefully improve with the results of ongoing research studies.

Given the risk of long-term consequences of repeated brain injuries, it is an open question as to the proper risk/benefit ratio for contact sports where there may be impacts to the head. These sports include football and boxing, of course, but also hockey, baseball, wrestling, and soccer. Professional sports players are more cognizant now about these risks, and organizations such as the NFL have been involved in research and education regarding these risks.

It is not clear, though, what to do at the school or college level regarding this issue. There are documented benefits of sports for children and adults, and increased fitness correlates with reduced chronic diseases such as hypertension or diabetes. On the other hand, as a society, we have to decide when the risks of repeated brain injuries outweigh the benefits of sports. There may not be one answer, as each parent or individual may have a different level of risk aversion or tolerance.

There may be various ways to minimize risk. Some amateur sports organizations have modified their rules to minimize head contact. Importantly, many organizations have begun more strictly following recommendations of the American Academy of Neurology that after a traumatic brain injury of any sort (including concussions), players should not be put back in the game; they should be cleared by a clinician before being allowed to play in future games.

New helmets have been produced, with sensors embedded inside to measure impact. Some helmets may also reduce brain impact after a hit through design and material improvements. Other technological improvements include better ways to assess on the field whether someone has had a concussion, such as computerized cognitive tests and measures of eye movement and balance.

It has often been said that prevention is better than a cure. That is certainly the case with repeated brain injuries. It is best to avoid additional brain injuries if possible. The number and timing may matter—a couple of concussions may be unlikely to cause long-term problems, but multiple concussions, especially in close proximity to each other, may be more concerning.

TAKE-HOME POINTS

Multiple concussions can cause more damage than a single concussion.

Symptoms following a concussion usually resolve on their own typically over a few weeks, but persons with multiple concussions may have long-lasting symptoms.

Accidents are not always preventable but extra caution should be exercised after a single concussion to prevent another concussion.

If you are having any issues after a concussion, get professional help immediately.

"When in doubt, sit it out."

Chapter 31

Future Treatments

Brain Stimulation
and Plasticity

In this last chapter, we discuss possible future treatments for brain injury, focusing on brain stimulation techniques—bringing us back full circle to our discussion of brain plasticity from early in the book. As you will recall, neuroplasticity is the ability of the brain to reconnect and reorganize; brain stimulation can facilitate this neuroplasticity.

Although not yet approved to be used in brain injury, brain stimulation techniques have been approved and used for a number of conditions to treat neuropsychiatric symptoms. Some brain stimulation techniques such as electroconvulsive therapy (ECT) have been in practice for decades, while others are newly emerging. Some newly emerging technologies include TMS (transcranial magnetic stimulation) and tDCS (transient direct current stimulation). TMS is currently FDA-cleared for a number of neuropsychiatric conditions, such as major depression, obsessive-compulsive disorder, and smoking cessation, while tDCS is not yet approved for clinical use.

All these brain stimulation techniques share the notion that the brain is dynamic and neuroplastic, and that by using electricity or magnetism, repeated stimulation of brain circuits can cause them to change over time.

The techniques utilize the power of the electromagnetic field, one of the critical fields in nature (other fields include the strong nuclear field, the weak nuclear field, and the gravitational field). A simple definition of an electromagnetic field is that it is something that is all around us created by electrical charges. Harnessing the electromagnetic field has led to almost all our modern technologies, including radio, television, Wi-Fi, computers, and cell phones. We are now at a point in history where we can use this incredibly powerful technology to affect our own brains.

The brain functions with both electricity and neurotransmitters. Much of what the brain does involves changes in electric potential and the subsequent firing of neurons. As neurons fire, they communicate with each other via neurotransmitters. As neurons repetitively fire together, they form connections together. According to the neuroscience maxim, "neurons that fire together wire together"; with brain stimulation, certain circuits are repetitively stimulated, causing the formation of connections and strengthening these circuits. Over time, it is easier for the neurons in these circuits to fire, and so they can more readily and efficiently perform their functions—that is what neuroplasticity is.

ECT, or electroconvulsive therapy, is one of the older brain stimulation techniques. ECT can be used to help control severe depression, bipolar disorder, or psychosis. ECT involves applying electricity to the brain directly. As the scalp acts as an impeder of electricity, a high level of electricity is needed to overcome this impedance and affect the brain. The level of electricity needed in turn causes a seizure. The whole goal of ECT, in fact, is to cause a generalized tonic-clonic seizure for a short period of time. A seizure is essentially (excessive) brain stimulation. Though it may be counterintuitive to think that such a practice is beneficial, it turns out that causing seizures repetitively over time in a controlled manner can cause significant neural plasticity–induced changes in brain circuits and can lead to dramatic improvements in depression, mania, or psychosis.

Since ECT involves inducing a seizure, the procedure must be done in a hospital setting and under anesthesia. The patient therefore needs to spend several hours in the hospital for each ECT session in order for the anesthesia to take hold and for time to recover from anesthesia. Given the anesthesia, someone must be available to drive the patient home. ECT can be thought of as potentially highly effective, but it is also invasive and can be logistically challenging. Patients with brain injuries have been given ECT, with good effect. Surprisingly, there are actually very few conditions that would absolutely preclude the use of ECT and could potentially be used with persons with brain injury. One noted side effect of ECT that can impact rehabilitation and functioning following brain injury is the effect it can have on memory, although most research studies suggest the memory deficits are temporary and associated with events around the time of the ECT procedure. Establishing risks and benefits becomes important when deciding whether ECT is an appropriate treatment.

An alternative might be TMS, or transcranial magnetic stimulation. Because TMS uses magnetism rather than electricity, the magnetic force goes through the scalp without restriction. The strength of the magnetic field used in TMS is usually the same as that used in magnetic resonance imaging (MRI) scans—1.5 tesla. The magnetic field causes targeted neurons to fire, and over time, neurons in the targeted circuits connect better and become more efficient in processing information and in their functioning.

TMS is less invasive than ECT and has a more desirable side-effect profile. It does not induce a seizure to cause its beneficial effects. There is no need for anesthesia and thus no need to be hospitalized; it can be done in an outpatient clinic setting. It does not cause cognitive problems, nor does it cause the potential cognitive harm and logistical complications of ECT. TMS also has the advantage that it is much more localized and focal than ECT, which allows more specific circuits to be targeted. However, we are still awaiting results of research studies to determine the types of TMS that are most effective in people with brain injury.

TMS is approved for major depressive disorder, OCD (obsessive-compulsive disorder), and smoking cessation by the FDA. Different circuits are targeted for different conditions: the dorsolateral prefrontal cortex in depression, the anterior cingulate in OCD, and the insula in smoking cessation.

In normal mood regulation, the dorsolateral prefrontal cortex modulates the emotional brain (particularly an area called the subgenual cingulate). Emotions allow us to respond appropriately to danger; however, our emotions must be calibrated to the situation. With major depression, sadness or lack of enjoyment is persistent and not necessarily calibrated to our external situation. The dorsolateral prefrontal cortex normally helps with this calibration, but it is underactive in depression. TMS strengthens the connections between the dorsolateral prefrontal cortex and the subgenual cingulate, or between the "cognitive brain" and the "emotional brain," allowing our emotions to be properly modulated.

In OCD, a circuit that involves the anterior cingulate is overactive. The anterior cingulate plays a role in terms of error detection. With excessive anterior cingulate activity, we may have a sense that something is wrong, that there is an error, even when there is not: this is what happens to people with OCD—obsessive thinking (repeated, persistent, irrational thinking that is distressing for the person) and then compulsions (rituals or behaviors to help manage these thoughts). Common obsessions include excessive worry about "germs," and a consequent compulsion could be excessive hand-washing. With TMS, the anterior cingulate is targeted to disrupt its functioning. Interestingly, TMS is not used by itself in OCD treatment. First, the person is exposed to something that elicits their obsessions and compulsions (such as being asked to touch a dirty garbage can if they have a fear of "germs"). This activates the anterior cingulate. Immediately afterward, TMS targets the anterior cingulate and disrupts this circuit.

Substance use disorders such as nicotine (smoking) addiction involve a circuit that includes the insula, deep in the brain between the frontal and temporal lobes. The insula is particularly involved in craving, which leads to further smoking. TMS for smoking addiction involves targeting the insula and the medial prefrontal cortex.

People living with a history of brain injury often have depressive and obsessive-compulsive symptoms, as well as substance use disorders (such as smoking), and given that TMS can work for these symptoms in the general population, it may work for them as well. However, there are not enough studies yet to suggest that TMS be used with brain injury. There have been both negative and positive studies. One note of caution is that those living with a brain injury may be more vulnerable to seizures (this is especially true if the individual drinks alcohol). Even though TMS does not generally cause seizures, some risk of seizure is still present. While this is not usually an issue in the general population, it may be more of an issue for those with a history of brain injury. TMS can be performed in such a way to minimize or eliminate seizure risk, but it is not clear if this method is as effective.

TMS might also be potentially helpful with cognitive disorders, such as attention and memory problems, which are common after brain injury. Current research programs are studying different forms of TMS and different target sites in the brain to help cognition. It may be that, like in OCD, a combination of therapy and TMS together may work best; in the case of cognition, the therapy would not be a behavioral therapy, but cognitive brain training. It may be that using cognitive brain training along with TMS in the same session may improve cognition, and this practice is currently being studied. TMS, which has the potential to be a game-changer in quality of life after brain injury, is thus still in evolution as a treatment for people with such injuries, but it is too early to recommend it quite yet.

Another brain stimulation technique known as tDCS (transient direct current stimulation) involves using a low electric current (one so low that it is hardly noticeable to the patient) on the scalp. tDCS is thought not to cause neurons to fire, but rather, nudge them toward firing. The premise is that, especially in combination with things like cognitive brain training, tDCS can encourage or influence certain brain circuits to fire more and thus connect more. tDCS is not yet FDA-approved for any condition. It is likely not as effective as TMS or ECT, but it is thought to be relatively low-risk. While some studies have shown potential benefit, we are still in early days in terms of the use of tDCS in brain injury. In the future, it is possible that it could be used along with physical and cognitive rehabilitation after injury.

A number of other brain stimulation techniques are in their infancy in terms of brain injury. Photobiomodulation is the use of red or near-infrared light to target the brain. Some data suggests that this technology could potentially improve mood and cognitive symptoms after brain injury. Deep brain stimulation (DBS) involves neurosurgeons placing electrodes in specific areas of the brain to help networks that have become dysfunctional due to brain injury. Preliminary data suggests potential benefit with DBS in brain injury. Vagal nerve stimulation (VNS) is FDA-cleared for major depression and epilepsy, but in this traditional form, it also involves neurosurgical placement. A new form of VNS called transcutaneous VNS (or tVNS) does not involve brain surgery; rather, it involves passing electric current across the skin of the neck; some data indicates potential benefit after brain injury.

In summary, brain stimulation overall is an exciting addition to our toolbox to treat neuropsychiatric symptoms. While it may be a bit early to use some of the techniques with individuals who have acquired a brain injury, it is still exciting that we are now able to use powerful technology to modulate brain circuits. There are ongoing research programs to assess TMS for PTSD, bipolar disorder, and cognitive impairment symptoms, and hopefully, we will be able to use brain stimulation to help these as well as depression and OCD symptoms in brain injury in the future. Since brain stimulation can be effective for any disorder where the brain circuitry is well known, in the future these techniques may also be used for other consequences of the brain injury (such as limb weakness after a brain injury caused by stroke).

TAKE-HOME POINTS

Although brain stimulation has been in existence for quite some time, there is an emerging understanding of its potential to enhance neuroplasticity, and new technologies to leverage neuroplasticity.

Transcranial Magnetic Stimulation (TMS) is now cleared by the FDA to treat major depression, OCD, and smoking cessation in the general population.

There is still ongoing research to refine brain stimulation strategies and make them available for clinical use, and they are not yet readily available for brain injury.

Epilogue

Leslie is a 41-year-old schoolteacher, a wife, and the mother of two young children. Her car collided with another car as she pulled out of the school parking lot one afternoon. Leslie was sober and wearing her seatbelt when she was hit. Paramedics found her unconscious at the scene of the accident, but she gradually regained consciousness by the time the ambulance arrived at the emergency department. A CT scan revealed contusions in the left side of the brain and a small bleed outside the brain (subdural hematoma), also on the left side. Leslie had sustained a moderately severe brain injury. The doctors opted not to do brain surgery. But Leslie developed weakness on the right side and had difficulty using her right hand and right leg.

Leslie received physical therapy (PT) in the hospital. Her doctors discharged her about two weeks after the accident, recommending that she receive outpatient physical therapy and that a neurologist and her primary care doctor monitor her progress.

Leslie continued with PT after her discharge, but she progressed slowly. Over the next few weeks, she also developed intermittent headaches, poor sleep, and fatigue, and she could not keep up with her responsibilities at the school. Leslie eventually had to take a leave of absence. She saw her doctors regularly and received treatment with various medicines for the headaches and insomnia. She returned to work three months after the accident, but even then, she felt that she wasn't efficient. She still wasn't driving, and she dragged her right leg a little—though her arm felt much better now.

As months went by, Leslie's husband noticed that she was sad, tearful, easily frustrated, and quiet. She was not spending time with the family; she came home from work tired and went straight to bed. About nine months after the accident, Leslie admitted to her husband that she just couldn't take it anymore; she needed professional help.

Together they consulted with her primary care doctor, who diagnosed Leslie with clinical depression and referred her to a neuropsychiatrist. The neuropsychiatrist confirmed the clinical depression diagnosis and saw Leslie regularly. He tried several different medications before he found a medicine that worked for Leslie. Meanwhile, he recommended that she maintain a timetable for the day, go to sleep and wake up around the same time every day, exercise for at least 20 minutes every day, and eat a healthy diet. He recommended some booster sessions of physical therapy to help her regain her strength, a few sessions of occupational therapy, and weekly sessions with a mental health therapist.

It took some time for Leslie's symptoms to improve, but after three months, she was doing much better. She felt better, she looked better, she had energy, and she found renewed inspiration for teaching her students.

We have had a long journey together over the course of this book, exploring the structure and function of the brain, the various ways brain injury affects the brain, how the brain can recover by using neural plasticity, and the emotional, behavioral, cognitive, and general neurological symptoms of the traumatized brain.

In this chapter, we synthesize what we have discussed throughout the book and summarize our recommendations. Our ultimate goal is to help you or the person you are caring for learn how to recover from the trauma of brain injury.

Leslie, in our opening story, is a patient of ours who sustained a moderately severe brain injury (a TBI) and developed depression after her injury. Her positive attitude, her compliance with the treatment plan, and the support of her family were all keys to her recovery. Her depressive symptoms resolved in a few months, and she was able to get back to her previous level of functioning. Everything that Leslie did is doable. We present her story to show that neuropsychiatric symptoms after brain injury are indeed treatable. Do not ignore them or be ashamed of them. Get help.

Leslie's story epitomizes what can be done to optimize outcomes in brain injury. Most importantly, Leslie was willing to accept what happened, and she did everything she could to recover. There is a trauma—a psychological trauma—when a sudden event occurs that upends our lives. Dealing with this trauma and accepting what happened is an important part of recovery for the traumatized brain.

Let's explore some of the specific reasons why Leslie's recovery went so well in the end. These are simple steps and techniques that you or your loved one with brain injury can also implement to help in recovery from brain injury.

Medical Records

Leslie brought all her medical records, including records of her hospitalization, to her first appointment with the neuropsychiatrist. Her records helped the doctor get a good understanding of Leslie's injury without having to speculate about what exactly happened in the accident and how severe her brain injury was. Having this information is valuable to a doctor, because many patients with brain injury do not remember the sequence of events right before, during, or after the injury. Having a record of Leslie's medical history and previous medications helped the doctor choose a medication that Leslie had not tried. Without these records, the doctor might have prescribed a medication that Leslie had tried before and that didn't help her, leading to inefficient care and further delays in her recovery.

The point is this: if you are caring for a person with brain injury, arrange for the doctors who are treating them to receive copies of all their medical records from the accident, as well as their full medical history, including all current and previous medications.

Medical Advocate or Companion

Leslie's husband accompanied her to most of her medical appointments. He was able to give a lot more information about Leslie's mood state and how it was impacting her, information that gave the doctor a better perspective on Leslie's illness. Because of the nature of mood, behavioral, and cognitive symptoms, the person with brain injury may have little insight into their symptoms.

The point is this: be sure that a responsible adult accompanies the person with brain injury to most if not all medical appointments, if possible. The medical advocate can take notes, answer questions that the person with brain injury may not be able to answer, and be aware of the doctor's recommendations for treatment.

Medication and Therapy Compliance

Leslie's compliance and willingness to follow recommendations served her well. She carefully followed the occupational therapist's recommendations for structuring her day and gradually building in new activities. She attended the physical therapy sessions and regularly practiced her PT exercises at home. She met weekly with the psychotherapist and used the sessions to grieve, discuss her losses, and accept her new deficit—the mild right-sided weakness. She also learned the importance of continuing to take her medications to keep her moods in balance.

The point is this: work with the person with brain injury to find ways to keep on track with treatment therapies and taking medications as prescribed. Enter all appointments on a calendar or day tracker that the person can refer to daily. Leave notes or reminders or set alarms to remind the person when to take medications.

These practices will serve anyone well. We provided tips in many of our chapters to help with specific conditions. Here we offer some general guidelines for recovery from a brain injury.

General Guidelines for Recovery from a Brain Injury

If you are a caregiver or family member of a person who is recovering from a brain injury, be supportive:

• Educate yourself about brain injury. Read, talk to professionals, or participate in a brain injury support group—a great venue for interacting with other people with brain injury and caregivers and families involved in the care of people with brain injury.

• Encourage the person you are caring for to seek professional help if you see that they are developing emotional, cognitive, or behavioral problems after a brain injury.

• Think safety first. If the person with brain injury shows or experiences a sudden change in mood, behavior, or cognition, or if the person becomes violent or aggressive, seek immediate professional help. Call 911 or emergency medical services if you believe anyone is in danger.

• Work with the person with brain injury to ensure that they are taking medications as prescribed and following all physicians' and therapists' recommendations. This can be a challenging task, but things will improve as you continue to work closely with the person who has suffered a brain injury. There is no formula or recipe for how to do this; you can find support and encouragement in working with someone who has expertise in this area (doctor, therapist) or interacting with someone who has similar experiences with brain injury (for example, attending brain injury support groups, discussing your issues, and getting feedback).

• Be creative; think outside the box. Brain injuries come in all shapes and sizes, and so do people. Don't be afraid to be unconventional in how you or the person with brain injury tackle challenges (one of our patients pinned a note to her shirt, upside down, so that she could look down and read it; that way she remembered to buy dog food at the supermarket on her way home from a physical therapy appointment).

• Reward or praise the person with brain injury when they do positive things and be sincere in your praise.

• Take care of yourself. Take breaks when you get tired or frustrated. You can't motivate the person with brain injury if you yourself are run down and feeling discouraged.

• Don't hesitate to ask others for help. Seek professional help if you are constantly feeling burdened and down. If you are having difficulties with your spouse or other family members, consider marital or family counseling. If you need a break, ask a trusted neighbor, friend, or family member to step in for a day or an afternoon.

If you are recovering from a brain injury:

• Educate yourself about brain injury. Start by talking to your doctor. Ask questions about the severity of your injury, the likely course it may take, and dos and don'ts.

• Protect yourself against a second injury. There are no guarantees in this world, but taking simple precautions, such as wearing a helmet if you are using a bicycle or motorcycle, wearing a seatbelt, and not driving under the influence of alcohol are prudent precautions.

• It is best to abstain from drinking alcohol or using illicit drugs. Even though marijuana may be legal in some states, the marijuana available on the street is not for your use, because you cannot know what other ingredients it contains. Labeling the percentage of the active ingredient is also not always accurate and consistent.

• Remember that working with a professional can help you gain a better understanding of your unique situation and teach you strategies to deal with your challenges. There is no reason to feel ashamed or embarrassed about getting help for these problems.

Hope for the Future

Having reviewed what we know now about how to get the best outcomes after brain injury, we want to share some promising future directions in the care of brain injury.

One advance that is now available to patients is pharmacogenetic testing. In this test, the doctor swabs the inside of the cheek and sends the cells to a lab for genetic testing. The tests reveal what genetic variants are in those cells that may affect the person's response to medications. For example, a person may have two versions of the "long" allele of the serotonin transporter, which might suggest that they are a good candidate for treatment with selective serotonin reuptake inhibitor (SSRI) medications. Pharmacogenetic testing also helps physicians determine which medications might work better based on how and how well a person metabolizes different medications. Pharmacogenetic testing has the potential to help with medication dosing and knowing which medications may be more likely to cause side effects. The indications, risks, and benefits of pharmacogenetic testing are still being worked out, but some physicians are currently using this test.

We discussed in chapter 31 the exciting possibility of using brain stimulation techniques to directly modulate damaged brain circuits. Breathtaking developments are still in the research stage with brain injury. But, now that we have learned more and more about the circuits of the brain and how mood, behavioral, and cognitive symptoms occur when these circuits are interrupted or damaged, we are reaching the point where it may be possible to manipulate brain pathways to improve symptoms.

All these research advances have great implications for those who develop psychiatric symptoms after brain injury. It is all the more important now that you or your loved one with brain injury realize what these symptoms are and not be ashamed to get help. As we have made clear throughout this book, these symptoms are real; they are not made up. There was a time, not too long ago, when some people may have doubted the reality of these symptoms. But no longer. Doctors and research experts in brain injury now appreciate more than ever the importance of treating emotional, behavioral, and cognitive symptoms that develop after a brain injury. Our knowledge and understanding of the neuroanatomy and treatment of brain injury is fast improving. Brain injury experts appreciate that emotional, behavioral, and cognitive symptoms can be related to the trauma just as much as such physical symptoms as weakness or loss of sensation in the limbs.

Our aim in this book is to help those with brain injury and their family members and caregivers understand their symptoms and how to improve them, as well as to teach people that psychiatric symptoms are real and directly related to brain injury. We are at the beginning of a landmark period in how we think about psychiatric symptoms; we are nearing the time when we can erase completely any lingering stigma still associated with psychiatry and mental illness. With this understanding, along with some support and hard work from family members and caregivers, persons with brain injury will recover optimally, in every sense of that word, from a traumatized brain. And perhaps even more than just recover—we can hope to use the power of neuroplasticity to heal the traumatized brain.

Acknowledgments

Our heartfelt gratitude to Dr. Peter Rabins for inspiring and motivating us to write this book. *The 36-Hour Day*, written by him and Nancy L. Mace, served as a foundation for this book.

We are much obliged and thankful to Joe Rusko, senior acquisitions editor of books on health and wellness, and Juliana McCarthy, managing editor, Johns Hopkins University Press, for their support and encouragement in helping us bring this book to fruition. Our very special thanks to David Goehring for his skillful review, excellent feedback, guidance, and edits, all of which helped to strengthen the book. This book would not have been completed without the guidance and assistance of this team.

To our patients and their caregivers, from whom we have learned most of what we know about emotional and behavioral problems following brain injury, we shall ever be grateful. We dedicate this book to them.

We are indebted and ever so grateful to Dr. Jessica McWhorter and Ms. Anastasia Edmonston for their meticulous review and tremendously valuable feedback. We sincerely appreciate the time and effort they took to carefully review each chapter and provide useful pointers, which were incorporated, and constructive criticism. Their input helped greatly to strengthen and shape the book. We thank them from the bottom of our hearts! Dr. Jessica Wolfman McWhorter is an assistant professor in the Department of Physical Medicine and Rehabilitation at Johns Hopkins School of Medicine and Ms. Anastasia Edmonston, MS CRC, is the coordinator of the traumatic brain injury partner grant project in the Older Adults and Long-Term Services and Supports Division at the Maryland Behavioral Health Administration, Maryland Department of Health.

In this book we provide specific suggestions for patients and family members. These are suggestions we make when we talk to our patients and family members. However, we would like to acknowledge the significant contributions made by other brain injury clinicians and researchers. This book is the result of our collective wisdom, and we appreciate the education and teachings we have had from our mentors and colleagues.

Our deepest gratitude to our families for their unconditional love and cheerleading as we worked on the book.

I would like to express my gratitude to my children, Shivum and Dhruv, for their wonderment about the nature of the world. I would also like to thank my wife, Deepti, for her consistent and pervasive support and encouragement. Without my parents, Vijay and Kirti Vaishnavi, I would not be in a position to have done this project, and so my eternal gratitude to them. Finally, my grandfather, Shyam Lal Vaishnavi, has always inspired me to investigate the nature of the brain and reality.

SANDEEP VAISHNAVI

I am incomplete without my family! My eternal gratitude and salutations to my parents, Mrs. Dhanalakshmi Devi Santappa and Prof. M. Santappa, for their bountiful blessings and unconditional love; to my husband, Narsima, my anchor and soulmate; to my children, Veena and Harsha, for giving me the strength and inspiration to keep moving forward; to Niketh, my son-in-law, for his constant support; to my grandchildren, Riya and Kiyara, for the insatiable joy they provide; and to my siblings, Shyla, Sunanda, Umesh, and Ravi, and their spouses, for their continuous encouragement.

VANI RAO

Glossary

aggression. Hostile, harmful, or destructive behavior that can be physical or verbal and can range from irritability to physical assault on others.

anomia. Difficulty in naming objects.

anxiety. An overwhelming sense of apprehension or fear.

apathy. A decrease in or lack of motivation.

aphasia. Disturbance of expression and comprehension of spoken language.

aprosody. Difficulty in appreciating or portraying emotions in speech.

arousal. The state of wakefulness that allows us to interact with the environment.

attention. Selection of one stimulus from the environment.

axon. A branch that extends from the soma or body of the brain cell. Axons send signals to other neurons.

blast injury. Injury that results from exposure to an explosion. Often encountered in the context of war or combat. Shock waves from the explosion damage the brain because of the sudden change in pressure brought on by the exploding device.

chronic traumatic encephalopathy (CTE). The developing concept that accumulated damage from a series of mild TBIs may lead to long-term impairment over the years.

circadian rhythm disorder. Disorders of the timing of sleep; for example, going to bed very early or very late or arising very early or very late.

clinical depression. A medical diagnosis describing sustained, persistent low (depressed) mood in a person who cannot enjoy usual activities and who may have physical symptoms in addition to depressed mood.

cognitive behavioral therapy (CBT). A form of psychotherapy that is based on the principle that thoughts and feelings influence a person's behavior. CBT trains the client to think more like a scientist, to examine whether the thoughts they are having are valid or supported by evidence.

complex partial seizure. A seizure in which the person feels an alteration of awareness, but the whole body is not affected.

computerized tomography scan (CT scan). An imaging technique that produces computer-processed X-ray images of cross-sections of the body.

contusion. Bruising of the brain.

coup-contrecoup injury. A common pattern of head injury in which brain damage occurs both at the site of impact (the coup injury) and on the opposite side of the head from the impact (the contrecoup injury).

delusions. Firm, fixed, false beliefs that a person has, despite evidence to the contrary.

dendrite. A branch that extends from the soma. Dendrites receive signals from other neurons.

dialectical behavioral therapy (DBT). A form of psychotherapy that focuses on distressing problematic behaviors and helps the client learn different, more rewarding approaches.

diffuse axonal injury (DAI). Damage to the axons as they are stretched in the back-and-forth movement of the soft brain within the bony skull in an accident.

divided attention. The mechanism by which the brain maintains focus on more than one task at a time.

electroencephalogram (EEG). A recording of the electrical activity in the brain.

epidural hematoma. A collection of blood right below the skull, between the skull and the dura mater, the outermost covering of the brain.

executive function. The ability to set a goal, initiate action toward the goal, monitor progress toward the goal, and modify the course if necessary to achieve the goal.

family therapy. A form of psychotherapy that focuses on the entire family and in which each family member participates.

generalized anxiety disorder (GAD). A medical diagnosis of persistent free-floating anxiety for prolonged periods that interferes with a person's everyday activities.

generalized seizure. A seizure in which the entire brain is affected, often leading to loss of consciousness and jerking movements throughout the body. There are many types of generalized seizure: tonic-clonic (also known as grand mal), clonic, atonic, myoclonic, and absence seizures.

grand mal seizure. *See* generalized seizure.

gray matter. A type of brain tissue that contains neurons.

group therapy. A form of psychotherapy in which a small number of people with similar issues meet regularly with a therapist to discuss their problems and discuss ways they have dealt with their problems.

hallucinations. Sensory experiences of hearing, seeing, feeling, or smelling things when there are no external stimuli.

hematoma. A blood clot or a collection of blood outside a blood vessel.

hemorrhage. Active bleeding.

illogical thinking. A pattern of thinking in psychosis in which thoughts are jumbled or disorganized; a form of psychosis.

impact injury. Injury that occurs when the head makes sudden, forceful contact with some object.

impulsivity. Acting on a whim without consideration of the consequences.

injury from inertial forces. Injury that results when the brain moves within the skull, but not as a result of impact to the head.

insomnia. The inability to fall asleep or stay asleep.

interpersonal therapy (IPT). A form of psychotherapy whose goal is to help the client improve interpersonal skills and either resolve or cope with interpersonal problems.

intracerebral hemorrhage. Bleeding within the soft tissue of the brain.

intracranial hemorrhage. Bleeding within the brain, either between the skull and the brain or within the soft tissue of the brain.

magnetic resonance imaging (MRI). An imaging technique that uses electromagnetic radiation to obtain pictures of the body's soft tissues.

mania. A state of heightened mental and physical activity.

memory. A collection of processes that lead to learning and recalling information.

narcolepsy. A condition in which the person experiences episodes of sudden and uncontrollable sleep.

neuromuscular junction. A synapse between a neuron and a muscle cell.

neuron. A brain cell; the brain's fundamental unit of operation.

neurotransmitters. Chemicals within the brain.

nonepileptic seizure. A type of spell that appears to be a seizure but gives no evidence of seizure on an EEG.

panic attack. A sudden wave of anxiety that occurs without warning. A panic attack can be so severe that the person experiencing it may think they are about to die.

partial seizure. A seizure that affects only one part of the brain, and there is not complete loss of consciousness.

penetrating injury. An injury sustained when an object penetrates the soft tissue of the brain.

post-traumatic stress disorder (PTSD). An anxiety disorder that develops after exposure to a stressful and traumatic event. The person with PTSD reexperiences the trauma in flashbacks or dreams.

psychosis. Both a mental and a behavioral disorder causing gross distortion of reality, disorganized emotional responses, and the inability to cope with ordinary demands of everyday life.

reticular activating system (RAS). A network within the brain that is responsible for consciousness, alertness, and awareness.

seizure. An abnormal amount of electrical discharge in either part of the brain or the entire brain that can produce body movements or thought disturbances or both.

selective attention. The mechanism by which the brain chooses which stimuli in the environment to engage with. It involves the ability to inhibit or ignore the processing of distractions.

selective norepinephrine reuptake inhibitors (SNRIs). Medications that increase the brain chemical norepinephrine. SNRIs are often used to treat depression.

selective serotonin reuptake inhibitors (SSRIs). Medications that increase the brain chemical serotonin. SSRIs are often used to treat depression.

sleep apnea. A condition of abnormal breathing while sleeping—usually a cessation of breathing while sleeping. Sleep apnea is associated with daytime sleepiness.

soma. The main body of a neuron (brain cell).

subarachnoid hemorrhage. A collection of blood closer to the brain than a subdural hematoma, but still outside the brain. Subarachnoid hemorrhages develop below the arachnoid mater, yet another membrane covering the brain, but beneath the dura mater.

subdural hematoma. A collection of blood between the brain and the skull, but below the dura mater. Subdural hematomas are closer to the brain than epidural hematomas, but still outside the brain.

sustained attention, or vigilance. The mechanism by which the brain maintains focus on something for a longer period of time than required for selective attention.

synapse. The space between any two neurons where chemical and electrical signals are transferred from one neuron to the other.

tonic-clonic seizure. *See* generalized seizure.

traumatic brain injury (TBI). A brain injury caused by physical trauma.

white matter. A type of brain tissue that contains nerve fibers, mostly axons that carry signals to different parts of the brain.

Resources

The following resources have been compiled for professionals as well as for individuals with brain injuries and their families by the Maryland Department of Health (MDH) Behavioral Health Administration (BHA), supported in part by grant number 90TBSG0060-01-00 from the US Administration for Community Living, Department of Health and Human Services, Washington, DC 20201.

Advocacy Organizations

Brain Injury Association of Maryland
biamd.org, 410-448-2924, toll free within Maryland, 1-800-221-6443

Maryland's BIAA affiliate offers information and referral services for individuals with brain injury, their families, and professionals. BIAM has a library of information and sponsors and holds an annual statewide brain injury conference for professionals, advocates, individuals with lived experience of brain injury, their families, and supporters.

National Association of State Head Injury Administrators
nashia.org, 301-656-3500

NASHIA's efforts are aimed at "assisting state government in promoting partnerships and building systems to meet the needs of individuals with brain injury and their families." NASHIA offers free information on a variety of brain injury–related topics including domestic violence, employment, and veterans. NASHIA also has many publications and webcasts on a variety of brain injury–related topics.

Brain Injury Association of America
biausa.org, 1-800-444-6443

The Brain Injury Association of America links callers from around the country to local resources.

Ontario Brain Injury Association
https://obia.ca/

Acquired Brain Injury Outreach Service
https://www.health.qld.gov.au/abios/asp/links
ABIOS, an Australian organization, has a brain injury website and resources.

General Brain Injury Resources

Behavioral Health Administration, Traumatic Brain Injury webpage
https://tinyurl.com/2p8aanrp
This page includes information and links to initiatives and products of Maryland's lead agency on brain injury. The Office of Older Adults and Long Term Services and Supports oversees these initiatives as well as the Federal TBI Partner Grant and the Maryland Brain Injury Medicaid Waiver. The page has links to fact sheets, brain injury screening tools, and professional training materials.

National Center on Applied Person-Centered Practices and Systems—Brain Injury Learning Collaborative
https://tinyurl.com/2p9h4ru9

Understanding Brain Injury: A Guide for the Family
https://tinyurl.com/5jfaafnv

New York Traumatic Brain Injury Model System, Mount Sinai Medical Center
https://tinyurl.com/rhm9br4k
Mount Sinai is one of the TBI Model Systems programs. It also houses the Rehabilitation Research and Training Center on Traumatic Brain Injury Interventions.

Administration for Community Living, Traumatic Brain Injury Program
https://tinyurl.com/4f8s4zb2
The Federal Traumatic Brain Injury Program is housed at the Administration for Community Living (ACL). This federal agency coordinates and over-

sees grants to states funded by Congress with the mandate to expand capacity of state systems to support and promote access to services for people living with a history of brain injury.

Centers for Disease Control and Prevention, National Center for Injury Prevention and Control

cdc.gov/traumaticbraininjury

The CDC offers information and educational resources for people living with brain injury, as well as medical professionals and those involved with youth sports.

TBI Model Systems Knowledge Translation Center

msktc.org/tbi

The TBI Model Systems Knowledge Translation Center is the repository of fact sheets on a variety of brain injury–related topics as well as information regarding the research findings of the TBI Model Systems Programs around the country.

Brain Injury and Behavioral Health Resources

Ohio Valley Center for Brain Injury Prevention and Rehabilitation

https://tinyurl.com/3c6jy93k

The Ohio Valley Center is one of the TBI Model Systems research centers. John Corrigan and his colleagues conduct research and publish on a variety of topics including TBI and substance abuse, domestic violence, and employment. Learn about the link between alcohol use and brain injury: https://tinyurl.com/29ezpvrj.

Learn how to screen for a history of brain injury as well as how to support individuals living with a history of brain injury: https://tinyurl.com/5bnk5v2u.

Traumatic Brain Injury and Substance Use Disorders: Making the Connections, toolkit for providers (2021)

https://tinyurl.com/mve97n7d

Client Workbook: Substance Use and Brain Injury (2021)
https://tinyurl.com/3yx49t6k

Substance Abuse and Mental Health Services Administration Advisory: Treating Patients with Traumatic Brain Injury (2021)
https://tinyurl.com/55wfdw4y

What Providers Need to Know: Behavioral Health and Brain Injury
ATTC Tip Card, SAMSHA Publication NO. PEP21-05-03-001, 2021
https://tinyurl.com/yu5mnkys

General Harm Reduction Resources

Center for Harm Reduction Services
https://tinyurl.com/msxwytkv
Information on harm reduction resources in Maryland, including naloxone and overdose prevention, syringe service programs, COVID-19 harm reduction guidance, and training and technical assistance.

Baltimore Harm Reduction Coalition and Maryland Harm Reduction
Action Network
https://baltimoreharmreduction.org/
Information on naloxone distribution, local overdose prevention advocacy, monthly training and wellness meetings, syringe services.

Employment Resources

Maryland Division of Rehabilitation Services (DORS) specialized services
for individuals living with acquired brain injury
https://tinyurl.com/2p8p78t2

Resources from the Disability Employment Technical Assistance Center
and the National Association of State Head Injury Administrators
(NASHIA).
Become a Champion for Employment! Guiding People with Brain Injuries

towards Work: A Resource for Supporting Individuals with a Brain Injury Continue or Pursue Work
https://tinyurl.com/2p8cz5v5
   You CAN Work after Brain Injury: Improving Your Employment Success
https://tinyurl.com/ypx73m69

Job Accommodation Network
askjan.org/media/brai.htm
   Provides useful articles dealing with employment after brain injury. Information can be obtained regarding individualized workplace accommodations and strategies that can be used to maximize success on the job. A service of the US Department of Labor's Office of Disability Employment Policy.

Understanding Brain Injury, a Guide for Employers
mayo.edu/pmts/mc1200-mc1299/mc1298.pdf
   Published by the Mayo Clinic and intended to provide an overview of brain injury and suggested strategies employers can implement to support those living with brain injury in the workplace.

Military Resources

BrainLine
brainline.org
   Website funded through the Defense and Veterans Brain Injury Center offers civilians, returning service members with brain injury, families, and professionals a variety of information and resources regarding life after brain injury.

Traumatic Brain Injury Center of Excellence (formerly the Defense and Veterans Brain Injury Center)
https://tinyurl.com/2rwrek7j
   An online resource from the Defense and Veterans Brain Injury Center is an initiative designed to promote traumatic brain injury awareness, education, and prevention.

Air Force Center for Excellence for Medical Multimedia
tbi.cemmlibrary.org
Offers a number of interactive tools related to brain injury, appropriate for individuals with lived experience, their families and supporters, as well as professionals.

Intimate Partner Violence Resources

Maryland Department of Health Behavioral Health Administration's Intimate Partner Violence and Child Malfeasance Resource Guide
https://bit.ly/3CrSGF6

Brain Injury Association of Virginia
biav.net/traumatic-brain-injury-domestic-violence

Resources from the Ohio State University and the Ohio Domestic Violence Network as well as a short video documentary on the relationship between brain injury and intimate partner violence:
https://tinyurl.com/y2nfnkb3
https://youtu.be/zp7uBCJ6Sko

US Government Accountability Office, June 12, 2020, report, *Domestic Violence: Improved Data Needed to Identify the Prevalence of Brain Injury among Victims*
gao.gov/products/GAO-20-534#summary
The report reviews the data available on the link between brain injury and resources available such as educational materials developed by the Ohio Domestic Violence Network for domestic violence service providers to support and screen individuals impacted by intimate partner violence.

Children and Youth Resources

Learn Net
projectlearnet.org/project_learn
This website, created by the Brain Injury Association of New York State, is geared toward children, parents, and teachers to help children with brain

injury navigate the classroom. Much of the information provided and strategies suggested are applicable for adults at home, in the community, and at work.

Colorado Kids Brain Injury Resource Network
cokidswithbraininjury.com
Although this website emphasizes resources in Colorado, there is very useful information for parents, professionals, and educators as well as a terrific educational animated video for school-age kids on how to take care of yourself if you experience a concussion.

Compiled by Anastasia Edmonston MS CRC, anastasia.edmonston@maryland.gov*, Maryland TBI Partner Project Coordinator, Maryland Department of Health (MDH) Behavioral Health Administration (BHA), updated 2022*

Suggested Reading

Nonfiction: For Medical Professionals

David B. Arciniegas, Nathan D. Zasler, Rodney D. Vanderploeg, Michael S. Jaffee, and T. Angelita Garcia, eds. *Management of Adults with Traumatic Brain Injury*. American Psychiatric Association Publishing, 2013.

Jonathan M. Silver, Thomas W. McAllister, and David B. Arciniegas, eds. *Textbook of Traumatic Brain Injury*, 3rd ed. American Psychiatric Association Publishing, 2019.

Nonfiction: For General Readers

Robert Cantu and Mark Hyman. *Concussions and Our Kids: America's Leading Expert on How to Protect Young Athletes and Keep Sports Safe*. Houghton Mifflin Harcourt, 2012.

Nonfiction: Firsthand Accounts of Life after Traumatic Brain Injury

Marilyn Lash. *When a Parent Has a Brain Injury*. Lash and Associates, 2012.

Trisha Meili. *I Am the Central Park Jogger: A Story of Hope and Possibility*. Thorndike Press, 2003.

Claudia L. Osborn. *Over My Head: A Doctor's Own Story of Head Injury from the Inside Looking Out*. Andrews McMeel, 2000.

Alix Kates Shulman. *To Love What Is: A Marriage Transformed*. Macmillan, 2008.

Carole Starr. *To Root & To Rise: Accepting Brain Injury*. Spiral Path, 2017.

Fiction: Living with Traumatic Brain Injury

Cathy Crimmins. *Where Is the Mango Princess?* Alfred A. Knopf, 2000.

Timothy Laskowski. *Every Good Boy Does Fine: A Novel*. Southern Methodist University Press, 2003.

Richard Powers. *The Echo Maker*. Farrar, Straus and Giroux, 2006.

Index

Page numbers in *italic* refer to illustrations; page numbers in **boldface** refer to tables.

HEALTH & WELLNESS BOOKS FROM HOPKINS PRESS

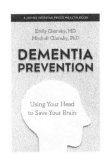 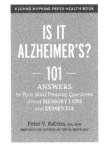 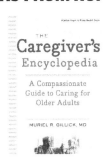 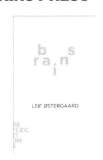

Dementia Prevention

Using Your Head to Save Your Brain

Emily Clionsky, MD, and Mitchell Clionsky, PhD

"A clarion call for taking action to reduce our risk of developing dementia and well-calibrated guidance on how to best improve our odds of staying cognitively sharp."
—Jimmy Potash, MD, Johns Hopkins Medicine

Is It Alzheimer's?

101 Answers to Your Most Pressing Questions about Memory Loss and Dementia

Peter V. Rabins, MD, MPH, best-selling author of "The 36-Hour Day"

"An excellent, accessible, and much-needed contribution to the popular literature. This highly approachable, usable book should be a resource for all those living with dementia and their families and caregivers."
—Cynthia R. Green, PhD, coauthor of *Through the Seasons: Activities for Memory-Challenged Adults and Their Caregivers*

The Caregiver's Encyclopedia

A Compassionate Guide to Caring for Older Adults

Muriel R. Gillick, MD

"An open conversation with a good friend who happens to know the questions you should ask and how to find the answers."
—Christine K. Cassel, MD, author of *The Practical Guide to Aging: What Everyone Needs to Know*

Brains

Leif Østergaard

A short but fascinating exploration of the brain and how this enigmatic organ is even more complex than we thought it was.

Reflections, a series copublished with Denmark's Aarhus University Press

 @JohnsHopkinsUniversityPress

 @HopkinsPress

 @JHUPress

press.jhu.edu

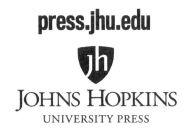